Healing
As Sacrament

Healing
As Sacrament

The Sanctification of the World

Martin Israel

Darton, Longman & Todd
London

First published in 1984 by
Darton, Longman and Todd Ltd
89 Lillie Road, London SW6 1UD
Reprinted 1985

ISBN 0 232 51580 8

British Library Cataloguing in Publication Data

Israel, Martin
   Healing as sacrament.
   1. Pastoral medicine   2. Pastoral psychology
   I. Title
   265′.82   BV4337

ISBN 0–232–51580–0

Phototypeset by Input Typesetting Ltd, London SW19 8DR
Printed and bound in Great Britain by
Anchor Brendon Ltd, Tiptree, Essex

It was there from the beginning; we have heard it; we have seen it with our own eyes; we looked upon it, and felt it with our own hands; and it is of this we tell. Our theme is the word of life. The life was made visible; we have seen it and bear our testimony; we here declare to you the eternal life which dwelt with the Father and was made visible to us.

(1 John:1–2)

Meanwhile our eyes are fixed, not on the things that are seen, but on the things that are unseen: for what is seen passes away; what is unseen is eternal.

(2 Corinthians 4:18)

Contents

Acknowledgement

Thanks are due to the publishers for permission to use material from the New English Bible, © 1970 by permission of Oxford and Cambridge University Presses.

Prologue

The ministry of healing is often disturbingly fragmented due to sectarian loyalties, each practitioner concentrating almost exclusively on his own small terrain in the vast field of wholeness. In fact, of course, the personality includes not only the physical body and the rational mind but also an insistent will to purpose that drives us on to our finest endeavour, that makes our lives ultimately meaningful in the face of the menacing approach of ageing, disease and death that conclude all mortal existence.

When our vision is extended to understand the ministry of healing as a sacrament of God's grace leading mankind to its proper place in the world, we can begin to grasp the meaning of complete human restoration in the divine image in which it is eternally created. This vision of restoration embraces not only humanity but also the whole of creation. It is with these themes that this book grapples, starting from what is known about man and his environment and proceeding to a vision of a restored cosmos in the divine image.

1

The Nature of Healing

As its most elementary and practical, healing can be defined as a restoration of health to a part of the body that was previously diseased. The body itself has a remarkable built-in system of healing whereby it can replace portions destroyed by injury or disease, prevent the invasion of organisms that take part in the various infections to which it is heir, and reject the ingrowth of foreign tissues. The discipline of medicine, especially the studies of physiology and pathology, is now in a position to shed much light on the many processes of healing whereby the body attains a normal state of function after a severe injury or disease. The one characteristic that soon strikes the observer is the remarkable order of the processes. There is a regulated outpouring of the cells and fluid necessary for healing both from the blood and the nearby healthy area, and when the end of healing has been attained the flow of fluid and the migration of cells ceases forthwith. Order and rhythm are features of the healthy body's functioning. Once order is disrupted and disorder predominates the disease becomes more serious; the most sinister is the unrestrained abnormal growth of cells that characterizes a tumour. This follows its own rules of growth, whatever they may be, and if it is malignant it will tend to destroy the whole organism in its relentless spread.

Medical science can describe these processes in terms of chemistry with ever increasing precision, but is still largely ignorant about the fundamental factors that initiate the chem-

2

ical response and control it. There seems to be a more subtle healing power that lies beyond the manifest phenomena of disease and healing than has yet been discovered by the biological or physical sciences. It appears to be related in some way to the emotional and mental life of the person, and this in turn is dependent on the meaning the person sees in his life and the purpose to which it is devoted. In any healing process there are factors involved that are strictly localized to the part of the body that is diseased. But there are also factors of a more generalized, or systemic, nature that seem to control the over-all response of the whole body to the assault of injury or disease. These include such tangible influences as diet and occupation, but there is also increasing evidence that mental attitudes are also of importance. The mind, itself intimately related to the brain, controls the body's response to many noxious stimuli that might otherwise destroy it.

The human personality functions on at least four levels – the physical body, the emotions that influence its actions, the rational mind that investigates and controls the environment on which life depends, and a deeper centre of moral decision which is traditionally called the soul. More acceptable contemporary names for this central focus of personality are the true self or spiritual self, which is to be contrasted with the ego self by which the personality expresses and asserts itself moment by moment in the environment. The ego consciousness fluctuates whereas the consciousness of the true self is stable; it defines the formed attitude of the person to the great themes of life: vocation, purpose, faith, dedication, renunciation and death. We are told by Jesus to love God with all our heart, soul, mind and strength and to love our neighbour as ourself (Mark 12:30–1). This means that all four functions of the personality have to be used in our devotion to God and his creatures. All four functions are to be properly, indeed perfectly, integrated so that they operate as a complete whole in unity as well as in diversity. It is this integrated action that is the basis of order, whether on the elementary level of the body's cells and organs or on the composite level of people and society. St Paul makes this very clear in his famous analogy of the various types of Christian believers

3

with the organs of a healthy body whose integrated whole is Christ himself. 'For Christ is like a single body with its many limbs and organs, which, many as they are, together make up one body. For indeed we were all brought into one body by baptism, in the one Spirit, whether we are Jews or Greeks, whether slaves or free men, and that one Holy Spirit was poured out for all of us to drink' (1 Cor. 12:12–13).

The basis of effective healing, by which I mean a healing made manifest by a changed attitude to life so that the local restoration of health becomes durable and progressive, is integration. The centre of integration is the spirit of the soul or true self, which informs the rational mind, cleanses and purifies the emotions, and renews the body with strength and vitality. Conversely, the state that precedes disease is disorganization of the body that is secondary to disintegration of the personality. This usually follows an emotional upheaval consequent on such disasters as disappointment, betrayal or bereavement. Our emotional life is especially close in its impact on the body; we all know the effects of anxiety or grief on the heart's action and the digestion, how the appetite is lost and the heart-beat is accelerated when we are in danger, and how all the body's functions are diminished when we feel unhappy and depressed. The emotions in turn are related to the state of the rational mind that determines coherent action in response to immediate exigencies or more distant need. But all are finally under the direction of the soul, which discerns ultimate purpose in the apparently meaningless flux of everyday life, a purpose that may indeed transcend the rational barriers of life and death.

It must be said, however, that even the most integrated person is liable to injury and infection, and if the injury is of massive extent the person will die at once. Similarly, an overwhelming infection can kill even a previously robust young person with dramatic speed. Nevertheless, in even such acute emergencies as these the individual tending towards integration of his personality is more likely to hang doggedly on to his life than his fellow with a diminished will to survive. When we consider the more chronic, long-standing conditions, the frame of mind of the person assumes an even more decisive role in the progress of the disease. As yet, we do not have the means to put these common clinical observations into a scientific framework with reproducible statistical data. This is because the progress of a disease and its tendency to recovery cannot be readily quantified in terms of such nebulous influences as the previous life-history of the patient and his dominant frame of mind. Furthermore, it is hard to compare the progress of diseases in a group of people with the differences in temperament and background that characterize each of us as a unique individual. Our response to life's various challenges is a very individual matter, a compound in fact of our conditioning and our unique personality. Nevertheless, despite these largely immeasurable factors, there is too strong a correlation between healing and integration of the personality to be dismissed out of hand as either a coincidence or a primitive superstition. Eventually, indeed, the person may learn to live with the affliction and transcend the limitations it exacts on his life. At that juncture the malady may so diminish in intensity that a slow, progressive healing shows itself despite all predictions to the contrary. In other words, the challenge of an apparently incurable disease may serve to integrate the sufferer's personality, after which a certain degree of improvement may show itself.

The radiance of a healthy body is an outer manifestation of the psychic energy that infuses and directs it. This vital energy that pervades the body and directs its inbuilt healing reserve has been tentatively called the *vis medicatrix naturae*, or healing power of nature. In days gone by it was heavily relied on by the experienced medical practitioner, who had comparatively little in the way of effective drugs to help him in his fight against the infection that was threatening the life of his patient. Quite often the support he was able to give with the simple therapies at his disposal saw the patient through the crisis of the disease and then to a slow convalescence which heralded a glorious return to health and activity. In this dramatic fight, I am convinced that the spiritual support given by the doctor was a major factor leading to his patient's recovery. This spiritual support need not have had a sectarian religious basis – though often it did in the more committed days of yore – for what it entailed was simply a giving relationship between the doctor and the person he was treating. When our own personal resources are integrated and mobilized on behalf of someone about whom we care very much, a powerful psychic energy proceeds from us to the source of our concern, and this seems to activate the natural healing force resident in that person. That subtle healing force, it would appear, stimulates chemical and other agencies in the body that set in action the various physiological processes which are geared to repel infection and reduce the effects of damaging factors on the body's metabolism.

We are indeed members of one body, to return once more to St Paul's analogy, and the healing force of its centre, which is Christ, extends to all its limbs and organs. This healing force is a property of the Spirit of God, that Holy Spirit who is the lord, the giver of all life. Without that Spirit there would be no life, and by his action there is growth of the individual into a healthy organism with an integrated personality that presages that ultimate state of coming to share in the very being of God. This last vision is expressed in 2 Peter 1:4, and there is added the promise of escaping the corruption with which lust has infected the world. In other words, healing is not simply an individualistic venture; it is involved in all human activity, indeed transcending the purely human realm of activity and pouring out from the Holy Spirit himself. Individual healing must always occur in a social context, inasmuch as the healing of society is a prerequisite for the total healing of the individual. On the other hand, it is the healed individual who alone is able to use his strength fully to assist the healing of society. Nor does society exist as an isolated unit; it depends on the world around it, deriving its nourishment and sustenance from nature. Therefore concern for environmental conservation and the welfare of all life are integral to a fully comprehensive view of healing. 'God loved the world so much that he gave his only son, that everyone who has faith in him may not die but have eternal life' (John 3:16). These familiar words define the whole Christian venture, that by the participation of the Son Jesus Christ in the entire pageant of life, that life may be redeemed from the slavery of sin, whose wages are death, and enter into the full thrust of eternal life. This entry is effected by the unhindered power of the Holy Spirit; who establishes his healing work

6

best in the person starting to lead the risen life with Christ. This life is one of prayer, service and sharing with all around him.

To mankind belongs the privilege and the duty of caring for the other inhabitants of our world, the animal and vegetable kingdoms. But man is also predatory on these lesser forms of life. What should have been a mission of service and conservation has all too often become an orgy of violation and destruction. In the Creation myth mankind and the animals thrive on the vegetation, but as the primal sin of self-regard at the expense of all other beings possesses man increasingly, so the idyllic harmony of the living world is disrupted and destroyed. After the Fall there is enmity between the serpent and mankind, which is followed by human animosity, recounted in the tragic story of Cain and Abel. Finally after the Flood, described in Genesis 6–8, God puts all animals into man's power for him to eat, provided he abstains from blood (Gen. 9:1–5). In this elaborate myth, a symbolic illustration of spiritual truth culled, no doubt, from actual events in the history of a primitive people, we see how a severance of obedience to God leads progressively to a breakdown in relationship between people, between animals, and eventually between all living forms. The one uses the other unmercifully for its own end, but none more cruelly and wantonly than man, armed as he is with immense intelligence and cunning.

St Paul says in Romans 6:20–3,

> When you were slaves of sin, you were free from the control of righteousness; and what was the gain? Nothing but what now makes you ashamed, for the end of that is death. But now, freed from the commands of sin and bound to the service of God, your gains are such as make for holiness, and the end is eternal life. For sin pays a wage, and the wage is death, but God gives freely, and his gift is eternal life, in union with Christ Jesus our Lord.

In the messianic age as seen in Isaiah 11:6–9, there will be peace and harmony among all the animals once more with a little child leading them. They will not hurt or destroy in all God's holy mountain, for as the waters fill the sea, so shall the land be filled with the knowledge of the Lord. When we

7

remember Jesus' statement that whoever does not accept the kingdom of God like a child will never enter it (Mark 10:15), this prophecy of Isaiah assumes renewed power. St Paul, in a vision of cosmic proportions, sees the universe itself freed from the shackles of mortality and entering upon the liberty and splendour of the children of God (Rom. 8:21). This is indeed the end of the spiritualization of all life in all dimensions of existence in the form of Christ's risen body. To me this is the true theology of healing. It commences on a simple individual plane, extends to involve human society, embraces all other forms of earthly life in its span, and finally takes in the whole created universe. Its paradigm is the resurrected body of Christ, at once individual to Jesus and yet at the same time communal for all creation, now raised from the corruption of death to the incorruption of eternal life.

All other healing is partial and incomplete even if it restores the integrity of a part or organ of the body to efficient function once more. Such healing, valuable as it may be in the short term, is all too liable to relapse if the individual continues on his heedless way, oblivious of the lesson his affliction should have taught him. Healing is not a patchwork repair; it is a re-creation of something that has strayed from the image that God originally conceived. It follows therefore that the suffering and pain that burden the dark events of our life, such as severe illness, redundancy, bereavement or betrayal, can be authentic healing agents in their own right. Anything that deflects a person from his previously heedless way of life and causes him to think, perhaps for the first time in his earthly career, about the deeper issues of existence is potentially an agent of healing. Sometimes we may, like the Prodigal Son, have to descend a considerable distance down the pit of despair before we can have the silent isolation in which to reflect in undisturbed clarity upon our past life. This may indeed be one reason why God sometimes says 'No' to our petitions for what we regard as healing and worldly success. Every experience in life bears its own lesson, and we will not pass by the barrier it erects until we have learnt how to transcend it. Every aspect of the personality has to participate in this process of growth and strengthening; no one part can be by-passed through excessive emphasis on another. The

8

criterion of effective healing is a harmonious balance of the personality, which in turn is an image of a balanced world in which people of different background, temperament and insight can work together as effective limbs and organs of one fully integrated body of mankind. This is indeed a sacrament of the Godhead beyond our knowledge and yet indefinably set in the centre of the soul of each person.

2

The Faith that Heals

Among them was a woman who had suffered from
haemorrhages for twelve years; and in spite of long treatment by many doctors, on which she had spent all she had,
there had been no improvement; on the contrary she had
grown worse. She had heard what people were saying about
Jesus, so she came up from behind in the crowd and
touched his cloak; for she said to herself, 'If I touch even
his clothes, I shall be cured'. And there and then the source
of her haemorrhages dried up and she knew herself that
she was cured of her trouble. At the same time Jesus, aware
that power had gone out of him, turned round in the crowd
and asked, 'Who touched my clothes?' His disciples said
to him, 'You see the crowd pressing upon you and yet you
ask, "Who touched me?" ' Meanwhile he was looking
round to see who had done it. And the woman, trembling
with fear when she grasped what had happened to her,
came and fell at his feet and told him the whole truth. He
said to her, 'My daughter, your faith has cured you. Go in
peace, free for ever from this trouble.' (Mark 5:25–34)

What is this faith that cured the woman with 'an issue of
blood' (in all probability from the womb, a complaint that
involved legal impurity according to the statute laid down in
Leviticus 15:25–7)? In the classical definition of Hebrews
11:1, faith is that which gives substance to our hopes, and

10

makes us certain of realities we do not see. This faith is not simply a vacuous wish for the unattainable; on the contrary, it is an active quality that works towards the realization of that which is desired, even if it does appear beyond attainment in terms of reason. The practical basis of an active faith as compared with passive wishful thinking is openness to the creative potentiality of life itself. This is the sole act of will that is necessary to start the growth into the fullness of being that God has in store for us.

This faith that heals does not demand an uncomprehending acceptance of theories, nor does it submit to the domination of powerful people who purport to special knowledge or charismatic gifts. It therefore does not demand suspension of the critical faculty of the mind. In this respect, it is important to understand that any way of alleged spiritual development that emphasizes one function of the person to the detriment or exclusion of another is fundamentally aberrant, indeed heretical. Balance and order are the essential qualities of all healing work that stems from the Holy Spirit, whereas imbalance and disorder have their end in chaos and destruction. Faith opens us to the immeasurable fecundity of God's grace, and its end is the perfection of the personality that shows itself in service of a type that we associate with the work of Christ.

There is a world of difference therefore between faith and credulity. Faith is an open, self-giving acceptance of an unknown, yet dimly glimpsed, purpose that guides the flow of the cosmos. Credulity is a sacrifice of the rational, critical faculty in order to follow blindly along a path directed by another person. The end of this path is bondage to the person who has led one or to the ideology that has captivated one's mind. Credulity is the price exacted by a human predator, of whom there are unfortunately representatives even in the world of healing, whereas faith is the mark of trust that is given as one follows the path that has been blazed by the saints of all the religious traditions; its end is a knowledge of God.

If we return to the healing episode that prefixed this chapter, we can consider the faith of the woman that led to her healing. She had for a long time placed her trust in the

11

established methods of the medical orthodoxy of her time, but had, if anything, become worse on this treatment. She had heard of the remarkable healing powers attributed to the young teacher from Nazareth, but had been chary of revealing the nature of her disorder to those around her because of the legal impurity associated with it. And so she suddenly opened herself unconditionally to the healing power of God as made available in the person of Jesus. To do this she required not only complete openness and trust, but also the courage to act, to step forward and touch the clothing of Christ. From this simple account we see that faith is consummated in two acts: an act of self-giving to God, however he may be conceived, and an act of commitment to follow the course his Spirit indicates.

When God hears our petitions, he does not automatically grant them, but if we offer ourselves, soul and body, as a living sacrifice before him, his Spirit will infuse us so fully that a change in our entire outlook is wrought. And this change penetrates to the very core of the personality, which is the soul, from which it proceeds to enliven and regenerate the mind, quieten and strengthen the emotions and heal the body. The healing is total, usually slow and progressive, but occasionally dramatically precipitate. On the whole, a slow, deliberate type of healing is ultimately more beneficial than a sudden, dramatic one. A sudden cure is liable to concentrate the whole attention on the body or the mind, depending on the nature of the illness. A slower return to health provides the sick person with more time to deliberate on his life's course, and to treat the healing he is receiving with sober reverence. That which comes to us far too easily seldom makes its impact permanently felt in the personality; after the initial rejoicing it tends to be taken for granted and forgotten. On the other hand, that which is accompanied by the sweat of the brow and the rugged toil of the hands acts as an agent of transfiguration of consciousness up to the level of caring shown by Christ himself. The healings wrought by Jesus were admittedly permanent – certainly there is no statement that any of those who were healed subsequently relapsed – but we must remember the nature of the person who performed the healing act. No one who came into contact with Jesus in a healing relationship could ever be as he was before. On the other hand, the outer healing was only the presage of a much greater, more important conversion that was slowly taking place inwardly.

When a person experiences conversion to Christ, his whole way of life changes. As St Paul writes, 'When anyone is united to Christ, there is a new world; the old order has gone and a new order has already begun' (2 Cor. 5:17). But that new order has to come to completion as the person's character is gradually cleansed of selfish desires, even the desire for his own life at the expense of another person. We know indeed that there is no greater love than this, that a man should lay down his life for his friends (John 15:13), but the practice of this supreme love that is also the final witness of a total healing comes late in our spiritual development. The early healings of the body and mind attested to in the ministry of Jesus are indeed sacraments, outer and visible signs of an inward and spiritual grace, of the complete change to be brought about in the whole person, so that he is resurrected to the divine life of Christ. Therefore the early bodily healings are not to be seen as ends in themselves but as the beginning of a new way of life in the person who has received them. The end of the Christian way is resurrection. When we consider how slowly even his disciples came to know Jesus and understand what he taught them, how they turned from him when he needed their support most urgently, and how long was their spiritual apprenticeship before they were worthy to receive the full downpouring of the Holy Spirit, we can see that Christ himself works quietly in the soul of a believer. A dramatic healing is to be understood both as an indication of God's eternal presence among us and as a special grace of encouragement bestowed on the humble follower on the way to full spiritual maturity.

The barrier to that faith which is a prerequisite for healing is not, paradoxically enough, doubt. Indeed, a faith that is not heavily overshadowed by doubt lacks earthly reality; it is liable to founder on the hazardous rocks of credulity on the one hand or be drawn into a destructive vortex of fanaticism on the other. In Mark 9:14–29 we have a dramatic story of a boy possessed of an evil spirit that produced recurrent fits.

13

The disciples were unable to exorcise the entity despite the power given to them by Jesus. Only he himself could perform this ministry of deliverance in this instance, so close was the destructive influence to the child. Only a person of supreme spirituality, one whose prayer and fasting (which typifies the ascetic life) brought him constantly close to God the Father, could deal with this demonic agency. But the most moving episode in this story is the frantic response of the boy's father to the statement of Jesus that everything is possible to one who has faith. 'I have faith; help me where faith falls short.' This is the faith that heals: a trust in the Almighty that is humble enough to know its own limitations, but nevertheless leads the person on in the obscure darkness where all judgement has to be suspended until the dawning of a new day. As one gropes in the shadows, so faith is given one until the light of fulfilment breaks through, and one's spiritual sight is clear and triumphant. The critical faculty now knows something that was previously hidden from its understanding: the mind as well as the heart and soul has been brought closer to divine reality. It should also be said that although modern medical science would immediately diagnose this child's complaint as epilepsy, a condition due to an aberrant neuronal discharge from the brain, it could still be possible that a malicious psychic influence was the trigger for the disordered activity of the brain in this particular case. We know too little about the interaction of body and mind through the brain to make any dogmatic statement about the matter.

The real barriers to a healing faith are arrogance and hostility. Arrogance is an aspect of a more basic sin, pride. This cannot yield its supremacy and domination to any person outside itself; it is in fact a denial of love, inasmuch as we love because God loved us first (1 John 4:19). The arrogant person puts himself out of reach of God's love, not because God ceases to love him but because he is not receptive to that divine love which moves the universe. Until the fall that inevitably follows pride, there can be no openness to God's healing power. Only then does humility appear; indeed, humility is the reverse side of the coin of faith. Humility receives God's love, and faith ventures out into the unknown in the power of that love. A variation of the theme of arrogance is demanding that healing should occur in a special way or believing that we deserve God's special providence because of our piety and work for his Kingdom. In the story of Elisha and Naaman the Syrian (2 Kings 5), humility and faith bring the powerful army commander to the prophet's door for healing of an unpleasant skin disease. But when Elisha simply sends him a message to wash seven times in the Jordan waters to become clean and healthy once more, he is furious. He expected the prophet to have made a show of spiritual power over him and to have invoked the name of God. He might indeed have forfeited his healing had not one of his own servants brought him back to his senses, bidding him perform the simple act that Elisha had prescribed. There are also some people whose very virtue stands in the way of healing, because they feel resentment that God should have treated them so badly. Until we move beyond all considerations of deserts and recompenses, and are open as a little child to God's grace, we will block the power of his Spirit in us.

God is not to be bribed; a person may in dire straits make a contract with God, promising certain works of charity and prayers provided that help arrives. Sometimes this agreement appears to work, but it is not due to God's partiality to that person. It is due to the person opening himself out to receive the Holy Spirit in faith. As his faith grows, so he will cease to relate to God on a basis of bargaining, but will instead attain greater communion with him at all times. The divine fellowship will be enough for him; all other benefits will fall into the background of his consideration. Even the righteous Job had to move from a concept of God as personal provider who has to be placated by suitable sacrifices, to one of a universal source of life who provides as much for the uncomprehending forms of nature as for the brilliance of mankind. Faith brings us to God, and good works follow in the wake of that relationship. The motivating force of those works is love, not fear or obligation, for no one who knows God can either fear him any longer, or feel obliged to obey him. Instead of any ulterior motive, there is self-giving service in love to him and all he has created.

15

Hostility is an absolute barrier to the healing power of God. It seems ludicrous to ask for healing and at the same time reject it. But the human mind is not infrequently divided against itself and all life. When Jesus went to his home town accompanied by his disciples and began to teach in the synagogue on the Sabbath, the large congregation that heard him was amazed. They wondered where he acquired his store of wisdom and how he worked his miracles, for they knew him as a carpenter and they were intimately acquainted with his family, none of whom amounted to much in the local society. So they fell foul of him, and 'Jesus said to them, "A prophet will always be held in honour except in his own home town, and among his kinsmen and family." He could work no miracle there, except that he put his hands on a few sick people and healed them. He was taken aback by their want of faith' (Mark 6:1–6). This lack of faith was an attitude of deliberate hostility to Jesus; the townsfolk were determined to cut him down to size, at least in their own estimation, and they succeeded in proving that there was nothing exceptional about him. But they were the losers, not he. God does not shower his gifts on us with profligate abandon. Though we cannot earn them, we have still to be ready to receive them gratefully and constructively. A humble and contrite heart is the chalice into which the divine grace pours most freely.

The person who is privileged to minister healing requires faith no less than the one receiving it. This faith is once more a trust in God's unquenchable mercy, not in one's own ability. The essence of a healing gift is an ability to relate rapidly and intimately to a large number of people. The relationship is not an intellectual agreement, but a psychic affinity. 'Deep calls to deep in the roar of God's cataracts' (Ps. 42:7). In the divine presence the souls of those devoted to God's love and ministering his healing establish a perfect relationship with those they are helping, and the Holy Spirit pours down on them all. The minister of healing should be a pure instrument of the Sprit of God, and this requires that the various blockages in the personality are dissolved by the love that comes from God. Peace of mind, openness to the fecundity of life's gifts, selfless service and a suspension of egoistic thought are the basis of the faith of all who give healing to others. Amongst the greatest obstacles to this ministry are an attitude of judgement in respect of the person being treated, a desire for personal acknowledgement, and an attempt to justify the ministry to sceptics so that they may be converted to one's own faith. Some practitioners place a failure to achieve a satisfactory result squarely on the lack of faith of the person they are treating. This in fact means a lack of faith in themselves: a failure diminishes their own self-regard, and this they cannot bear. It is a terrible thing ever to accuse a suffering person of bad faith; this judgement belongs to God alone. Those who are psychically attuned can sometimes sense a resistance to healing on the part of the patient comparable with the rejection that Jesus experienced in his home town, but it is prudent not to reveal one's impression directly. Instead, undemanding love may slowly erode and break down that resistance with patience and forebearance.

As long as one wants personal triumph, the Holy Spirit is excluded from one's work. The essential attitude is 'Yet not what I will, but what thou wilt' (Mark 14:36). It is, I firmly believe, God's will that there should be universal healing, but the way is his, not ours. When we interpose our desires in the process, we deflect or even block the power of the Holy Spirit, and if anything, we delay and prevent healing taking place. In the spiritual life, it is a general rule that the harder we try the less we achieve. In no area of spirituality is this more true than that of healing. When we try we are asserting our ego, which invariably looks for results to inflate its sense of importance. When we are quiet in contemplation, a higher wisdom can infuse us; this wisdom subdues the claims of the little ego and allows the spiritual power of the soul to be concentrated and properly directed. As Jesus teaches, 'Whoever cares for his own safety is lost; but if a man will let himself be lost for my sake and for the Gospel, that man is safe' (Mark 8:35). As we give of ourselves to God in simplicity and trust, so he fills us with all good things. It is thus that the Holy Spirit works to his best advantage. We are not primarily concerned in extending our faith to others – this again is the work of the Holy Spirit. What we are here to do is simply to give unreserved love to all who will accept it. It was thus that Jesus proclaimed the good news that the kingdom of God was close at hand. In the end our faith in the goodness of life and the love of God is transmitted in the silence of blessing to those around us who are groping for some meaning in their disordered lives.

It is noteworthy that little children and animals frequently respond very well to healing, whether by prayer or by direct physical contact in the practice of the laying-on of hands. Their openness is limitless since they are uncontaminated by the deepening stain of worldly guilt and personal resentment. It is indeed true, as Jesus taught, that whoever does not accept the kingdom of God like a child will never enter it (Mark 10:15). But the second act of faith that we have already noted, a commitment to follow the course that the Holy Spirit reveals, cannot be within the range of a child, let alone an animal. The same would apply to a person receiving intercessory healing prayer at a distance and unaware of it; perhaps he would be so ill as not to be able to respond rationally even if he were told that prayers were being offered for his healing. The answer here lies in the commitment of those who have requested healing for their offspring or their pets, or who have appealed for help for someone at a distance who is seriously ill. The commitment of those seeking help for someone unable to respond directly provides the necessary impetus for the Holy Spirit to start his healing work. As in the instance of infant baptism where the commitment of the parents and godparents is a very important part of the sacrament, so the concern of those who ask for healing on behalf of a third party plays its part in effecting a cure or at least an amelioration of the trouble. The hope remains that a rational being may take on the commitment of another's caring when he returns to health. Certainly the harvest of deep intercessory prayer has included many previously indifferent people who have subsequently been brought into an active, progressive faith.

Faith is tested sometimes by apparent rejection. Jesus at first rejected the appeal of the Syro-Phoenician woman that her daughter might be delivered from an unclean spirit. He said to her provocatively that the children (of Israel) should be satisfied first; it was not fair to take the children's bread and throw it to the dogs (the Gentiles). But she replied that even the dogs under the table eat the children's scraps. This gesture of supreme humility confirmed the faith she had in the power of Christ, and as a consequence her daughter was delivered from the troublesome entity (Mark 7:24–30). Commitment to God is an essential ingredient of the faith that saves. Had the woman been so affronted by the rebuff she had received that she turned away in resentment, there would have been no healing. Jesus certainly reveals himself in a hard, rather uncompromising, light in this episode, though I am convinced there was a subtle sense of humour concealed beneath the façade of indifference he displayed to the Gentile woman. In everyday life the apparent rejection is repeated whenever our prayers for healing are apparently unheard by God despite our previously irreproachable behaviour. We have to persist; patience is another ingredient of faith. Even when there is no apparent outward change, we are still being renewed inwardly for the great trial ahead of us. Everything Jesus said and did was in preparation for his death and passion, and for the initiation of his disciples to full spiritual mastery. Faith transcends the demands of the personal self, or ego. In its fullness it embraces the world in selfless devotion.

This chapter commenced with a reflection on the healing of the woman who had 'an issue of blood', but in fact that was merely an episode in an even greater story, the raising to life of the daughter of Jairus, the president of one of the synagogues (Mark 5:21–43). Jesus was summoned by her father when she was at death's door, but his faith in the healing power of Christ was absolute. It is recorded that while Jesus was still speaking to the woman who had been healed by touching his cloak, the news came of the death of Jairus' daughter. Jesus, however, told Jairus not to be afraid, but only to have faith. When he arrived at Jairus' house, it was clear that the child was dead, but Jesus, accompanied by his three closest disciples Peter, John and James (who were also to witness both the transfiguration and the agony at Gethsemane), approached the motionless child and resuscitated her. We may, armed with modern knowledge about states of suspended life bordering on death – so-called clinical death – dispute whether the child was really dead or not, but it is quite apparent that Jesus performed a miracle in that she immediately arose and walked about. Jesus infused the child with the Holy Spirit who is the lord and giver of life, and she revived to continue her work in the world before she, like the remainder of mankind, was to be called to a timely death and resurrection to a new form of life. Again the faith of her father played its part in assisting the work of Christ. He was a loving intercessor between God and his afflicted daughter. Perhaps the three disciples were present to perform a similar role; alternatively they were privileged to see a physical resuscitation in order to augment their own faith, which was, as later events in the life of Jesus were to show, less perfect than they had believed.

It is interesting that the child was twelve years old, and the woman had suffered from haemorrhages for twelve years. Twelve is the sacred number of the Bible: twelve were the sons of Jacob, the tribes of Israel and the apostles of Christ. In the book of Revelation (7:4) we read that from all the tribes of Israel there were a hundred and forty-four thousand who had received the seal of God upon their foreheads, twelve thousand from each of the twelve tribes. They were to be saved from destruction. In the case of both the woman who was healed and the child who was brought back to earthly existence from physical death, the period of twelve years can with profit be seen to represent a time of purification in the world. The woman had gained faith through prolonged physical suffering and was at last ready to be healed. The child was to be lifted above a superficial earthly consciousness to a cosmic view of reality, such as is repeatedly described by those who have been clinically dead, during which time they have had a near-death experience of transcendence. Both the woman and the child had entered a new life; they had in fact received a fleeting glimpse of resurrection as the old order passed away and a new life unfolded before them.

3

The Act of Contrition:
Repentance and Healing

When after some days he returned to Capernaum, the news went round that he was at home: and such a crowd collected that the space in front of the door was not big enough to hold them. And while he was proclaiming the message to them, a man was brought who was paralysed. Four men were carrying him, but because of the crowd they could not get him near. So they opened up the roof over the place where Jesus was, and when they had broken through they lowered the stretcher on which the paralysed man was lying. When Jesus saw their faith, he said to the paralysed man, 'My son, your sins are forgiven'.

Now there were some lawyers sitting there and they thought to themselves: 'Why does this fellow talk like that? This is blasphemy! Who but God alone can forgive sins?' Jesus knew in his own mind that this was what they were thinking, and said to them, 'Why do you harbour thoughts like these? Is it easier to say to this paralysed man, "Your sins are forgiven", or to say, "Stand up, take your bed and walk"? But to convince you that the Son of Man has the right on earth to forgive sins' – he turned to the paralysed man – 'I say to you, stand up, take up your bed and go home'. And he got up and at once took his stretcher and went out in full view of them all, so that they were astounded and praised God. 'Never before', they said, 'have we seen the like'. (Mark 2:1–12).

If faith in terms of openness to God is a prerequisite for his Holy Spirit to infuse us and bring us to wholeness, a like openness to our deeper selves, that which borders in fact on the unconscious mind, is necessary for the power of the Spirit to penetrate to the depths of the personality. Amongst the superficial blocks in faith are, as we have seen, pride, hostility, and resentment. A deeper and more pervasive hindrance is the guilt that clouds our peace of mind and prevents us being fully receptive to the love of God on which our very existence depends. Until we have come to terms with the guilt that lies deeply in the soul of all rational creatures, we cannot be fully open to God's love for us: his love is always available, being constant and unconditional, but we all too often occlude its full impact by closing the shutter of the mind in self-deprecation born of feelings of unworthiness.

Guilt is the subjective response to the fact of sin. 'For all alike have sinned, and are deprived of the divine splendour' (Rom. 3:24). St Paul adds that we are justified – brought into a right relationship with God – by God's free grace alone, through his act of liberation in the person of Christ Jesus. Our guilt deprives us of the divine splendour, and only when we seek pardon, which is in fact free to all who are humble enough to ask it, can we re-enter the full healing relationship with God. The proof of God's grace lies in the assumption of sin by the Son, Jesus Christ, so that he is with us in our agony and brings us with him to his resurrection, a presage of which occurs in the sacrament of baptism.

To many contemporary thinkers the very concept of sin is outmoded. What was once regarded as sinful behaviour is now seen to be a reaction against the authority exerted against us by the powerful figures of our childhood, especially our parents and teachers. This conditioning, which is an inevitable part of our education to full adulthood, can undoubtedly assume a dictatorial role that stultifies the full flowering of the personality. The Freudian super-ego is formed by such a constellation of authority figures that leave their permanent impress on the unconscious. In this way any action that contravenes the criteria of acceptability laid down by the super-ego brings with it a feeling of guilt that can cripple one's will and thwart the journey towards self-actualization.

Another feeling of guilt may follow one's departure from the well-known beaten track of a conventionally acceptable life to a hidden destination devoid of the assurance of comfort. To quit one's peer group on economic, political or religious grounds not only leads one into a wilderness of ostracism but also fills one with a feeling of having betrayed those previously close to one; indeed, the feeling of betrayal is probably projected psychically on one by those whom one has left. Guilt feelings have therefore to be confronted directly and analysed rationally. They may be rooted in frank sin, as we shall see, or else they may be merely childish throwbacks of which one must be relieved and disembarrassed, often with the help of a counsellor or psychotherapist.

But there is a third source of guilt also, one that is related to one's present behaviour and one's treatment of other people. This applies especially to the betrayal of colleagues and the casual discarding of those no longer of use to one. It can be called existential guilt, a guilt that derives from one's actual relationship with the world around one. There is a central focus in all of us which we call the soul, or true self. This is the seat of an innate morality that determines human behaviour and choice of a level higher than merely selfish acquisitiveness based on such rudimentary demands as nourishment, shelter, and physical comfort and security. This innate morality recognizes elementary justice, of which even a small child is acutely aware. If it is unfairly accused or deprived, there is, as it were, a raw area inside its personality that cries out for the balm of justice, and its pain will not be assuaged until that justice is forthcoming. In the parable of the importunate widow and the unscrupulous judge (Luke 18:1–8), the callous judge eventually attends to the widow's complaint in order to get relief from her constant pleas for justice. So long as the core of the personality is in distress and its sore rankles, there will be a central disruptive focus that will wreak havoc on the rest of the person – body, mind and emotions. The two events in our lives that injure the soul directly are an injustice done to us and a sin we have committed against another person. Personal injustice that is not remedied leads to a resentment that in due course may warp the entire personality. Personal sin that is not acknowledged and confessed leads to a guilt that puts the person progressively out of communion with all people, and not only those he may have actively injured: so close is human solidarity that to have hurt one person is to have assaulted the whole community. In terms of the parable of the sheep and the goats (Mat. 25:31–46), what we failed to do to another person, however humble, we failed to do to Christ also.

It is incidentally in this context that we are told not to fear those who kill the body, but cannot kill the soul, but to fear him rather who is able to destroy both soul and body in hell (Mat. 10:28). Unrelieved resentment and unforgiven guilt damn the soul. Whether the soul can ever be finally destroyed is doubtful, since it, like the body, is God's gift to us. But it may experience unmitigated hell until it, like the Prodigal Son, comes to itself in its abject misery and calls for help. Thus all those who sow the seeds of hatred in others, especially the purveyors of vile propaganda that sets members of one race, religion or social class against their fellows of a different background, are especially to be feared. The bodily destruction that may follow in the wake of organized hatred is nothing as compared with the injury sustained by the soul both of those who perpetrate the outrage and those who suffer under it.

The soul, furthermore, cannot be brought to health by purely psychological means. Divine grace alone can exorcise the spirit of resentment on the one hand and guilt on the other. But competent psychotherapy can bring the person much closer to receiving the unconditional love that comes from God. To begin to face one's past life and present difficulties in the presence of another person is the beginning of healing, for it requires a basic humility even to come to someone else for counsel. Indeed, the sacrament of penance – the confession of one's sins before a priest and the granting of absolution that follows it – is a most powerful healing aid. I doubt whether there can be any effective healing, and by this I mean one that is progressive and persistent, until the person is cleansed of his guilt and resentment so that he can be fully open to God's grace.

When our consciousness is blocked by guilt we cannot face ourselves or those around us. Until we have opened ourselves to God in humble confession, the block remains and the Holy Spirit in all his power is denied us. This denial, I repeat, is due to our own recalcitrance and not the judgement of God, whose nature it is always to have mercy. The act of confession and the absolution that always follows it reconciles man to God, for God was in Christ reconciling the world to himself (2 Cor. 5:19). But can resentment be confessed and healed? After all, guilt accrues from our own past sinful actions, whereas resentment is the attitude that injustice evokes in us. On the surface it is quite justifiable to feel aggrieved when we have suffered an injury due to the evil actions of another person. The effect of these actions may leave a permanent mark on our personalities – a scar, as it were, on our souls – and although the very ground under us may cry out for justice, as Abel's blood did from the ground in which it was shed (Gen. 4:10), recompense still seems never to be forthcoming. In this respect one thinks especially of the countless millions who suffered hell in prison camps in this present century. The great majority died, and they carry on their work in the life beyond death. But what of those who remained alive and had to sustain themselves in this world? Can they ever come into right relationship either with God or with their fellow men?

Resentment itself is as destructive as guilt. It rapidly assumes the continuum of a vicious circle and leads the person in its grip to the very depths of hell. There are three possible means of escape from this downward spiral: a realization of the many benefits one still enjoys despite the wounds of the past, an appreciation that one's own life prior to the tragedy was far from perfect – in other words that one too has had a sinful past – and the devotion and ·love of those around one. Of these, the last is the most immediately pertinent. One can begin to unburden oneself of one's misery to someone who really cares – and that person must have traversed his own valley of darkness before he can understand sufficiently to be of help. That person, like the Suffering Servant of Isaiah 53, can bear another's sufferings and endure his torments. The resentment of the afflicted one can flow into this counsellor, and the process of healing can be initiated. At this point there can be a realization of personal guilt, so that instead of crying out for justice there is instead a humble confession of sins and a call for general forgiveness. Then at last the person becomes open to God and can perform the supreme act prescribed by Christ: love your enemies and pray for your persecutors (Mat. 5:44). This approach, it must be stressed, is very different from the detached 'forgiveness' advised by social theoreticians who reduce all personal responses to economic or psychological conditioning. To forgive fully one must have experienced an inner hell that has been illuminated by the unconditional love of God, a love fully shown in the perfect sacrifice made in his life by Jesus himself. Then, and then alone, is one so changed that God can work and speak through one. In other words, forgiveness, that is always of God, can issue authentically only from the lips of the person who has experienced the forgiveness of God; the test of that forgiveness is a changed personality, one that no longer seeks personal recompense but instead gives of itself totally to the service of its fellows. In the passage of Scripture that prefixed this chapter, the lawyers rightly disputed Jesus' right to forgive sins, but they did not understand the divine prerogative of the one who gave the absolution. When we have received the forgiveness of our sins, we in turn are qualified to forgive those who have sinned against us. If we still cannot forgive a person who asks our pardon, we have not yet opened ourselves fully to God's love. On the other hand, we cannot fully forgive someone who does not acknowledge his evil actions until we are so caught up in the love of God that the life we live is no longer our own, but the life that Christ lives in us (Gal. 2:19).

We should never be ashamed of our feelings, however naked they may be. The end of the spiritual life is not their suppression but their transfiguration. Our emotional reactions to the hurt that we may have received – or of greater pertinence, to the wrongs done to other, more vulnerable people – must be acknowledged and given free rein in our imagination. Here they can cause no harm to others, while at the same time they are released from the censorship of the unconscious mind, where they would otherwise be confined. While unconscious they have immense psychic potency to cause internal damage. On the other hand, once they are released into full consciousness they cease to be agents of subversion that may lead to psychosomatic diseases or even serious moral lapses (in an attempt to get their own revenge on other people whom they wrongly identify with those who caused the trouble originally). Once we have wreaked our punishment on those who have done wrong in the safe confines of a vivid imagination, we can see the end of such destructive fantasies and return to a mature consideration of the circumstances of the case. Then we will cease to long for revenge and seek more for healing, both of ourselves and those who have acted wrongfully. It is in this context that Jesus' words from the cross, 'Father, forgive them, they do not know what they are doing' (Luke 23:34), find their most profound significance.

Is disease the result of sin? Often there is no direct relationship. The diseases of children are surely not the consequences of their past guilt. On the other hand, I have little doubt that disease in itself is a result of cosmic disorder. If there were no sinful attitudes in the world, it seems certain that disease and death as we know them would show a completely altered complexion. When we return to the myth of the Fall in Genesis 3, pain, suffering and death followed in the wake of human disobedience to the divine spark present in the soul of mankind. This is co-eternal with the transcendent God who is far above his creation but intimately involved in its unfolding. This tendency to sin is hereditary, no doubt a corollary of the free will given to men and women by God; without free will there might be no danger of doing wrong, but the reverse side of the coin would be an inability to give of oneself in love. The infant seizes instinctively its mother's breasts, but there is no love in that action. Years later, perhaps only when it has attained independent adult stature, it may grasp the sacrifice and love that have been expended on its nurture and education. Only then does the child begin to love its parents, and in so doing it also acknowledges all those who live in selfless devotion to their fellow creatures.

Nevertheless, even if an illness is not caused by a special sin, our generally sinful attitude that has shown itself in the various unpleasant actions we have committed in the past, prevents us being fully open to the healing power of the Holy Spirit. Until we have come to terms with our incomplete attitude to life and to those with whom we live and work, we will not be completely healed. The practice of recollection each night, when we are about to retire to bed, is a very powerful spiritual exercise and a compelling prelude to our final prayers before dropping off to sleep. In the words of Psalm 51:3–4, 'For well I know my misdeeds and my sins confront me all the day long. Against thee, thee only, I have sinned and done what displeases thee, so that thou mayest be proved right in thy charge and just in passing sentence.' If we transgress the law of life we suffer accordingly until we put ourselves in right relationship with God once more by humble confession. It is not as if we are telling God anything new to him: what we are doing is to make our sinful inclinations fully open to ourselves in the divine presence, so that there is no cavern of subterfuge into which we can hide from the realities of our past life. Then, if the will is chastened and ardent, it can be strengthened by the Holy Spirit, and a new directive to our life is ordered. In confession, before a priest, the priest himself is a sacrament, being the outer, visible sign of the inward, spiritual grace of God. His personal concern is an outflowing of the love of God by which all healing is effected. His blessing prefigures the new life to which we are directed and into which we are welcomed. But we must play our part, else even worse may befall us.

The essential penance that should follow absolution is one that strengthens the will, so that the penitent may be in a stronger position to repel temptation in the future. The best self-mortification is the giving of oneself to other people, especially those one has wronged, in devoted service. Even if those against whom we have sinned are now no longer alive in the flesh, we can still repair the damage we have done by remembering them in our prayers and serving their brothers – who are those around us wherever we may be – in caring dedication. If I have done a good deed to even one person, I have done it to Christ also (Mat. 25:40). Inasmuch as Christ is universally present as the stranger on our own road to Emmaus, a good deed performed to any person is a gift to all humanity. And in this action of selfless service I begin to identify myself with all people, in this way passing beyond the tyranny of the ego with its constant demands and complaints, and entering into the full consciousness of the soul. In soul consciousness there is no barrier to the inflow of the Holy Spirit, so that I am at last in unrestricted access to the full thrust of that Spirit.

As we have already noticed, St Paul says, 'When anyone is united to Christ, there is a new world; the old order has gone, and a new order has already begun' (2 Cor. 5:17). The person who has confessed his sins in contrition and self-dedication to God and the world, is a sacrament of the one to be who has moved from the old order of attrition and death to the new order of union with God and with his fellow men. He is an earnest, a foretaste, of the new man resurrected in the likeness of Christ. As St Paul writes at the end of his passionate letter to the Galatians, 'Circumcision is nothing; uncircumcision is nothing; the only thing that counts is new creation' (Gal. 6:15). When we return to the great penitential Psalm 51 and read the words, 'Create a pure heart in me, O God, and give me a new and steadfast spirit' (verse 10), we see how this miracle of re-creation follows an act of true contrition and an opening forth of the self to God's unquenchable love in childlike faith. Then at last the inflow of God's healing Spirit can proceed unhindered, and a re-creation of the whole personality may be initiated.

It is interesting that in the spiritual way the essential barrier to faith is not doubt but pride, an attitude of mind that is so sure of its own rectitude that it will not allow itself to be available to new possibilities of God's self-revelation. In the same way, the great barrier to forgiveness is not a crippling awareness of guilt but an overweening sense of self-righteousness that is made rigid in resentment. So long as I cannot forgive others, including life itself, for my present misery, I will remain in dark isolation with myself as my only god – and what an impotent god that is! But as soon as I can yield my self-righteous stance and gaze with compassion at the creatures around me – including those who have injured me – I can glimpse my need for forgiveness no less than theirs. But whereas I at least can acknowledge that need and fling myself on the ground before God in abject prayer, those who have abused me remain in dark ignorance about themselves and what the future life has in store for them. Psalm

73 expresses perfectly the fate ahead of the unrighteous man who achieves worldly prosperity: he is set on slippery ground and is being driven headlong into ruin; his end in a moment is dreadful, cut off root and branch by death and all its terrors (verses 18–19). This is the great advantage that the innocent have over the guilty, no matter how much they may have suffered at the hands of the wicked.

But the matter does not rest there. Once the innocent have mastered their resentment and have also felt the need for final absolution, their blamelessness is transfigured by the forgiveness of God into love. No longer do they look for justice, let alone revenge. Instead they turn their thoughts and gaze to all who have wronged them, and seek to be the instruments of their forgiveness also. Love works unremittingly for the redemption of all that is imprisoned in hatred, fear and ignorance. It can never rest until all its brothers – all God's creatures – are free to receive the life-giving power of the Holy Spirit. Therefore the saints of this world and the next work ceaselessly for the healing of all that is perverse, unclean and imprisoned in chains of resentment and fear. The teaching of Jesus that we should pray for our persecutors (Mat. 5:44) is the way of our release from any remaining pangs of resentment no less than their liberation from the bonds of past wrongful attitudes that have caused them to act destructively to their brethren. In Christ we no longer look in eager anticipation for the downfall of the wicked as an end in itself. While the cry for justice is as strong as ever, it is seen to be merely the first stage in a universal redemption from sin, of which we are all partakers no matter how virtuous we may consider ourselves. It is followed by a prayer for all men that they may cease to sleep in the ignorance of materialistic illusion and awake to the glory of the spiritual reality that upholds and sustains the material universe. Only then can the sacramental significance of every mortal action be grasped: everything we do and say in love and healing at this moment is a sign of God's resurrected world in eternity.

4

The Refashioning of the Will

Later on Jesus went up to Jerusalem for one of the Jewish festivals. Now at the Sheep-Pool in Jerusalem there is a place with five colonnades. Its name in the language of the Jews is Bethesda. In these colonnades there lay a crowd of sick people, blind, lame and paralysed. Among them was a man who had been crippled for thirty-eight years. When Jesus saw him lying there and was aware that he had been ill a long time, he asked him, 'Do you want to recover?' 'Sir,' he replied, 'I have no one to put me in the pool when the water is disturbed, but while I am moving, someone else is in the pool before me.' Jesus answered, 'Rise to your feet, take up your bed and walk.' The man recovered instantly, took up his stretcher and began to walk.

(John 5:1–9)

There can be no healing until the sick person wants to be healed. This does not simply mean that he should have no hostility to the one who ministers to him, remembering how hostility blocks absolutely the healing power of the Holy Spirit. It means that the afflicted person's will must be directed positively and unequivocally to the path of recovery: he must desire healing with his undivided heart and mind. But what is this will that Jesus challenged in the man who been crippled for so long? The man would surely have protested his desire to get well if he had been challenged at

31

any period of his illness. It is easy enough to make glib affirmations of an almost self-evident type, for who would not want to become healthy again after a long period of infirmity? But the heart is the most deceitful of all things, desperately sick and almost unfathomable (Jer. 17:9). Indeed, the very concept of a free, autonomous will is dismissed out of hand by many psychologists and social scientists, for they know how imprisoned our responses are in emotional turmoil, adverse conditioning from our earliest years, and the economic environment in which we have had to battle for survival. Yet if we have no personal freedom to choose a particular direction of progress, our lives become increasingly meaningless so that eventually there is no future ahead of any of us other than immediate sensual stimulation and superficial conviviality.

It is true that our actions are powerfully influenced by our environment. This includes the conditioning we had initially to undergo from the earliest period of our life onwards as part of our training to become socially acceptable, useful citizens. To it is added the group solidarity that is exacted as a price for our acceptance as members of our particular niche in society. Nevertheless, there is an inner spark in us all that responds to the ultimate values of existence. These can be summarized in the concept of integrity, which unites the platonic triad of beauty, truth and goodness into a composite whole. That which offends against aesthetic taste in the world of art, intellectual truth in the realm of learning, and goodness (or love) in human relationships strikes at the heart of the personality in which the spark of the soul, called the spirit, eternally burns. 'The light shines on in the dark, and the darkness has never mastered it' (John 1:5); this statement is true as much of the spirit in all of us that is our point of contact with God as of God incarnate in Jesus who blazes the trail of truth and love to his own death. He says to Pilate, 'My task is to bear witness to the truth. For this I was born; for this I came into the world, and all who are not deaf to truth listen to my voice' (John 18:37). It is from the point of truth in the depth of our personality that the authentic will emanates. It is free yet directed by the Holy Spirit to fulfil itself to its perfection.

Freedom necessitates choice. In the words of Deuteronomy 30:19: 'I summon heaven and earth to witness against you this day: I offer you the choice of life or death, blessing or curse. Choose life and then you and your descendants will live.' In the service of God there is perfect freedom, for we can be ourselves without shame or the need for justification when we give of ourselves in childlike faith to him. He knows us far better than we know ourselves, and because his nature is love, he accepts us as we are. Provided our will is directed to his service – and this enlightened will is the action of the spirit, which is the central core as well as the animating force of the personality – he raises us up to something of his own stature seen in the person of his Son, Jesus Christ. It is the will deep in us that is the outer manifestation of the soul's action. It determines whether we remain slaves to the world's demands and our own conditioning or whether we respond to a nobler calling: to follow the path ahead of us that leads to a fulfilment of our personality in Christ.

Let it be said at once that not all conditioning is deleterious, nor are all the world's demands a hindrance to our development as fulfilled people. Without the training and teaching imposed on us during the formative years of our youth, we would not be able to cope with the society in which we are obliged to live and work. Without the assistance provided by the world around us we would not be able to survive for any length of time. Furthermore, not every impulse that comes from the soul is necessarily healthy; the spirit cannot err, being one with God, but the soul is a fallible agent. It learns in the hard school of life the essential lessons of humility, faith, sacrifice and love, so that eventually it places itself under the direct guidance of the Holy Spirit who comes to its own spirit. Balance and order are the bases of all healthy living: the demands of society have to be integrated with the thrust of the personal will, so that our own fulfilment as people may be set in equilibrium with our duties to those around us. This is indeed the immediate purpose of life as well as its final end. It follows that in the end we have to be detached from all outer clinging for assurance and security, and find the centre within us from which the will can choose freely and definitively. In many people's lives, the will lies dormant until some dramatic, often cataclysmic, event demands an immediate conscious response. Then the will initiates the full reasoning process, guided always by the intuition, and a choice is made. This is one that may determine the future direction of the person's life: there may be a conscious opting for life rather than death for the first time in his experience, for the usual state of many of us is that of a sleep-walker until we are jolted to consciousness by the threat of destruction.

Why should one not wish to be healed, assuming there are no ulterior motives, such as the sordid attraction of financial compensation or sheer laziness? To be healed means that one has to return to the world once more and bear one's own responsibilities. One can no longer live in a shaded light where one can hide from the demands of society. In the healing act that prefixed this chapter, once the cripple had accepted Jesus' ministry, he at once became a centre of controversy. It happened that he was healed on the Sabbath, when the Law proscribed any activity other than worship. This carrying of his bed on the Sabbath immediately put him beyond the pale of religious convention, and he had eventually to name the person who had healed him (John 5:10–15). At once he became a focus of disturbance in the community because of his association with the controversial teacher and minister of healing, Jesus of Nazareth. No longer could he lie concealed in the shadows of non-commitment. As he gave of himself to health once more, so he had to stand up and be counted: was his ultimate allegiance to God, made manifest in Jesus, or to the comfortable security of the community, ruled over by a theocracy of priests and doctors of the Law? To be associated with Jesus was to be put in fear of one's life, as Peter was to discover some time later: he chose a thrice-repeated denial of his Lord to the possibility of accompanying him to the cross. And then he came to himself and wept bitterly for his own private betrayal of his true nature, mirrored in Jesus Christ. Only then did the will of Peter show itself free and vibrant, as he dedicated the remainder of his life to following his Lord and giving of himself to all who would receive Jesus.

Health is ultimately in our own hands. God gives freely to

all who seek, but we have to contain the gift and use it constructively. Once we have given of ourselves to God, a new way of life opens to us. Its three demands are prayer, service, and sharing with others. We can no longer lead the old thoughtless life of self-indulgence and unawareness of the needs of others; regression is tantamount to death.

Jesus was no sentimentalist. He spoke out directly against hypocrisy and dishonest dealing. In the instance of the cripple whom he had healed, Jesus warned him, now that he was well again, to leave his sinful ways, lest he suffered something worse (John 5:14). In this respect his teaching about the danger of re-infestation by an unclean spirit is especially apposite.

> When an unclean spirit comes out of a man, it wanders over the deserts seeking a resting-place, and finds none. Then it says, 'I will go back to the home I left.' So it returns and finds the house unoccupied, swept clean, and tidy. Off it goes and collects seven other spirits more wicked than itself, and they all come in and settle down, and in the end the man's plight is worse than before.
>
> (Mat. 12:43–5)

Whatever views one may have about the obsession of the personality by outside psychic forces – and it is wiser to have an open attitude to the possibility rather than to dismiss it out of hand as a relic of pre-scientific superstition – it is certain that until the person has attained a degree of wholeness, which is of a different order to a mere cure of some disability or disease, one trouble is bound to follow another. It may first be an illness that is alleviated by drugs or surgery, which is followed by an accident causing bodily injury. This may in turn be succeeded by an emotional or mental breakdown, or some financial disaster, or a betrayal in a deep personal relationship. Furthermore, these misfortunes may not simply befall one personally, but be visited on one's family also. Until there is a shift in basic perspective, a change in heart (or metanoia) in fact, one trouble will follow another as surely as night follows day. And the person will quite plausibly curse his bad luck or else attribute the manifold misfortunes to God's inscrutable punishment. In fact

35

the punitive consequences of thoughtless actions are brought about by the spiritual law of life that is transgressed only at our own peril. Without this basic law which is enshrined in the moral teachings of all the great religious traditions and reduced to their essence in the two commandments of Christ – the love of God and of our neighbour as ourself – there could be no communal life. When each individual is for himself alone, there can be little place in his scheme of survival for anyone else apart from his immediate family. Each wars against the other until everyone is finally destroyed. No one group is self-sufficient, nor will others accept a role of permanent bondage to those with greater immediate power at their disposal.

All this is obvious enough on a social level but we often do not apply it in our private lives. Until we have the time to reflect on our past attitudes in our present distress, and pray humbly for forgiveness and a strengthened will, we will not be healed of our disabilities. When Jesus told the cripple he had healed to leave his sinful ways, he was urging him to adopt a way of life that transcended his past selfish attitude: he was told to give more to others as he in his turn had been given new life by Christ. To whom much is given, much is expected. The fees charged by a competent doctor are a fit reward for his expert help in relieving distress and restoring function to a previously disabled part of the body. By contrast, God charges no fees at all for his supreme healing work: ours is the donation to make. If we give nothing, we will relapse into ill-health. But if we give nothing less than ourselves to him, we will move from death to life of a new dimension in which our greatest joy will be to bring health to others. It is a law of the spiritual life that stagnation invariably proceeds to regression into old, destructive ways of thought. Conversely, the movement forward in faith is the only way of progress to the new life of the future.

It is nevertheless important to acknowledge that the unaided human will is more likely to lead to destruction than to a renewed life. Acting on its own, the will cannot move the personality out of the rut of past conditioning. The more we believe we are changing our way of life, the more obvious it is to the outside world that we are merely altering certain superficial approaches while deep down within there is the same selfish, fearful personality at work. Therefore the human will must be infused with the divine power that flows to it in the person of the Holy Spirit. In other words, the fallible, rather crude, native will is spiritualized through the action of prayer. In prayer we bring ourselves by a willed effort to the heavenly grace of God; this we cannot grasp but only seek in self-giving faith. But, as Jesus reminds us, to knock is to have the door opened, to ask is to receive, and to seek is to find (Mat. 7:7–8). In prayer we are filled with God's love and infused with his Spirit. Our will is spiritualized – indeed a foretaste of the spiritualization of the whole personality at the end of time – and then we can do the work that God has set before us. This is to collaborate with him in the re-creation of the world in the image of Christ. God needs us in the sustenance of our world no less than we need him; the proof of this divine grace is shown in the incarnation, when the Word itself became fully flesh and dwelt among us. It was to the end that we might bear witness in our transformed lives to his presence that he came to us and participated fully in the human pageant of glory and suffering.

For the will to be incisive and clean in its action there has to be a progressive opening-up of the whole personality. The unconscious part where the debris of the past lies concealed has to be brought to the light of day where it can receive the word of life and be healed. When Jesus was baptized by John, then alone did the Holy Spirit descend fully on him in preparation for the great ministry ahead. But that same Spirit led him, not immediately to the heights of glory but first to the valley of darkness. In the wilderness he remained for forty days tempted by Satan. He was among the wild beasts; and the angels waited upon him (Mark 1:12–13). The wilderness is the darkness of unenlightenment, of ignorance, which surrounds the earthly consciousness of mankind. The prince of the unredeemed world, Satan, governs that consciousness whose watch-word is, 'For me first'. What happens to the others is at most of marginal concern. Though without sin, Jesus became intimate with the sinful environment that envelops our world. There was nothing in man's nature that was foreign to him, so close was his psychic empathy to mankind and his spiritual nature to his Father. The forty days are, of course, symbolic of a long period of time – in fact his entire ministry on earth. The wilderness experience culminated in passion, crucifixion and a descent into hell, so that no depth of human despair was left untouched by his presence, no person too insignificant or evil to have escaped his concern and identification. It could in truth be said of Christ's ministry that by his wounds all wounded people are healed, an exact reproduction of the life and death of the Suffering Servant, portrayed in Isaiah 53.

All this has to be repeated as an interior experience in the lives of those who are striving towards a total healing. The cause of a failed healing is often ambivalence in the basic attitude to life: one half of the person wants to move onwards and scale the spiritual heights while the other half prefers the seductive comfort of inertia. If the will is not active, the attractions of the *status quo* will triumph over the urge to move on in life. As Jesus says, 'No one who sets his hand to the plough and then keeps looking back is fit for the kingdom of God' (Luke 9:62). It is the unresolved complexes in the unconscious that especially act as agents of subversion, deflecting the full attention and commitment of the person to travel onwards towards completion. They speak seditiously in the language of fear, resentment, defeat and failure if any new venture is proposed. It is this aspect of self-deprecation and doubt that is especially baneful to any further progress in the path of life. Doubt about the claims of others is the seed of wisdom; doubt in the rightness of one's own movement towards healing is the darkness of death. The life moving towards that salvation which is the measure of true healing is one of self-denial in the service of God; this service shows itself in self-giving to the neighbour in distress who, as the Parable of the Sheep and the Goats demonstrates, is the unknown Christ constantly with us as we traverse our own road to Emmaus. 'Anything you did for one of my brothers here, however humble, you did for me' (Mat. 25:40). The Emmaus road was one of pain and disillusionment to the bereft disciples until they noticed the stranger on the way and took him into their company. They did not know at first who that stranger was, but they were able to say, with hindsight, after the Master had revealed himself to them at the breaking of the bread, 'Did we not feel our hearts on fire as he talked with us on the road and explained the scriptures to us?' (Luke 24:13–32).

The will that has entered into the darkness of the unconscious and has brought to the light of day all that obstructs the power of God from working the fullness of his healing within the personality is also the will that leads the person to the beatific vision. The way to heaven is always through hell, for the vital reason that the way to God is one that redeems and heals all fallen elements on the path. In the economy of God all is sacred, no matter how far it may have fallen from its pristine glory in the perversion wrought by human nature. We cannot rise to God until we have taken all that appertains to us along with us and brought it to the throne of the heavenly grace. And then comes the miracle: the sordid article of earth is seen to be a sacrament of God's glory. It becomes a sacrifice worthy of the highest praise.

No one who enjoyed Christ's fellowship could escape his searing scrutiny. He was no liberal sentimentalist or condoner of any action other than the highest. But the perfection he represented was that of God working within the soul of the individual sinner, for he saw the divinity that lay within the meanest members of his society, typified by the prostitutes and the venal tax-gatherers. When we read of God's jealousy for his people Israel, God was not concerned about himself and the constant rejection he received during their frequent periods of apostasy. He was concerned about them and the betrayal of the highest within them they so often wrought by their treacherous disregard for the Law and the life it demanded. This jealousy is similar to that of a parent who guards the reputation of its child during periods of temptation and insult. In order to fulfil itself and its charge, that parent will not flinch from disciplinary action: 'for those whom he loves the Lord reproves, and he punishes a favourite son' (Prov. 3:12). Therefore we are told not to spurn God's correction or take offence at his reproof.

Healing requires the entry of the whole person into a new way of life, in which the seductive ease of the past is sacrificed in favour of service for all creatures in the future. If even one part of our desire is for the allurements of self-indulgence, we will remain anchored to the past. There can be no forward movement that does not encompass the whole of the personality. And this is the essential human dilemma, so often repeated in the history of ancient Israel as recounted in the Old Testament: the earnest will to follow God's commandments was invariably betrayed by the seductive attractions of the present scene. The essential need of man is commitment; the 'lower nature' of the body is committed to physical comfort and security which find their fulfilment in the acquisition of money, the forging of advantageous social and professional relationships, and the grasping after power. The 'higher nature' of the soul, informed by the spirit within, lies all too often in complete abeyance. It is made to feel something of an unnecessary, if not unwelcome, intruder in the path of assurance devised by the intellect and pursued by the body. But what does it profit a man if he gains the whole world at the expense of his soul? This terrible question is posed in one way or another by all the great world religions, but by none more starkly than Jesus himself (Mark 8:36). The whole world is an ephemeral illusion if it is divorced from the spiritual love that sustains and transfigures it. Until there is a commitment to the life that builds and sanctifies, the person himself remains confined to the darkness of futility and mounting fear, because all that is tangible in this world is also mutable and destructible. As Jesus tells his disciples, 'You must work, not for this perishable food, but for the food that lasts, the food of eternal life' (John 6:27).

It must finally be emphasized that in the person attaining integration there is only one nature, the full personality facing the uncreated light of God where it is transfigured into his likeness from splendour to splendour (2 Cor. 3:18). The body is lifted heavenward to partake of the intimations of immortality that surround it, in contrast to which the attractions and comforts of this world are merely ephemeral sensations. The soul, at the same time, incarnates more deeply into the flesh so as to learn the mighty lessons of service and renunciation in the limitation of a time–space milieu. The body teaches the soul some vital lessons of availability and punctuality, while the soul progressively transfigures the body from a purely animal structure to a spiritual vestment of finest quality through which the whole world can be charged with spiritual power. In other words, both the lower and higher natures are of God, and when they are integrated in obedience with the divine will, they bring nearer the promise of resurrection of the whole person into something of the measure of Christ.

To return finally to the man who was paralysed for thirty-eight years and unable to enter the pool at Bethesda in time to avail himself of its healing power, we see in him the paradigm of the previously uncommitted person who has unconsciously taken refuge in ill-health. His healing by Christ shows us not only a bodily cure, but also a strengthening in inner resolve with a renewed mind and a refashioned will. He is a sacrament of the total person re-created in the likeness of Christ, now responsive to God and responsible in his actions to serve all those around him as he once was served in his infirmity.

5

The Unobstructed Vision

As he went on his way Jesus saw a man blind from his birth. His disciples put the question, 'Rabbi, who sinned, this man or his parents? Why was he born blind?' 'It is not that this man or his parents sinned,' Jesus answered, 'he was born blind so that God's power might be displayed in curing him. While daylight lasts we must carry on the work of him who sent me; night comes, when no one can work. While I am in the world, I am the light of the world.' With these words he spat on the ground and made a paste with the spittle; he spread it on the man's eyes and said to him, 'Go and wash in the pool of Siloam.' (The name means 'sent'.) The man went away and washed, and when he returned he could see. (John 9:1–7)

This healing episode starts with an account of the restoration of sight to a man who was blind from birth. It continues, as in the case of the man who had been paralysed for thirty-eight years, with an encounter with the Jewish authorities who once again objected to the healing because it was done on the Sabbath. The man and his parents were minutely cross-questioned, because most of the doctors of the Law regarded Jesus as a sinner and were already plotting against his life. Eventually in exasperation the man who had been healed says, 'All I know is this: once I was blind, now I can see'. In the end he was expelled from the synagogue, another

example of how the healing wrought by God brings the individual into open controversy where he can no longer be mute,
but has instead to take a definite stand in the name of truth.

In this healing miracle the blind man attains spiritual
enlightenment as well as physical sight. The religious authorities, on the other hand, sink deeper into spiritual darkness
because they refuse to face the light of God, wilfully closing
their minds to its impingent rays. They remain spiritually
blind even though their physical sight remains unimpaired.
Jesus puts this tragedy into stark relief when he says to some
Pharisees in his company, 'If you were blind, you would not
be guilty, but because you say "We see", your guilt remains.'
In the same context he says, 'It is for judgement that I have
come into this world – to give sight to the sightless and to
make blind those who see' (John 9:39–41).

The portals of our inner vision that looks upon and
comprehends a deeper purpose to the manifold changes of
each passing moment, are, in our natural state, all too often
blocked by the cares and distractions, the material and psychical debris of the world around us. The scales of material
striving and emotional desire will continue to occlude our
deeper sight so long as we are immersed in worldly consciousness, in which we equate the trees of selfish, individualistic
endeavour with the wood of ultimate fulfilment. Often the
shadow of an imminent crisis looms so large in front of us
that it assumes the proportions of an unscalable mountain,
and we retreat in disarray before the menace of the unknown
without even having the courage to assess its demands from
a distance. Our view of reality is distorted by the narrow
range afforded by the ego-conscious vision in which we norm-
ally function, and many of the blockages we encounter are
created, and certainly magnified, by the uneasy ramblings of
an unstable mind. We see in another person often what we
project of ourselves on to him; only when we have been
liberated from our ego-directed field of vision can we see him
as an individual in his own right. Then for the first time we
may encounter kindness and consideration in one whom we
had previously categorized as cold, snobbish or dictatorial.
There can be no healing until we see life truly and of a piece.
Then, at last, we can participate in that life in full dedication,

giving our own unique essence to it for its greater glory as well as our emancipation from the bonds of selfish desire, whether they be a concern that others should think well of us or the expectation of recompense for our work.

'Where there is no vision the people perish' (Prov. 29:18). A more modern translation of this famous aphorism substitutes the words 'break loose' for 'perish'. When the mind is not focused on a teaching of high spiritual potency, the entire personality begins to vacillate in its purpose, and it is soon captivated by the glamour of meretricious trifles. Inevitably the person wanders off distracted and proceeds aimlessly; he soon encounters the various monsters that inhabit the dark verges of unfrequented paths. Jesus says, 'The lamp of the body is the eye. If your eyes are sound, you will have light for your whole body; if the eyes are bad, your whole body will be in darkness. If then the only light you have is darkness, the darkness is doubly dark' (Mat. 6:22–3). The will itself is of little avail if it lacks guidance. Only the light of God within can be a sure guide into the darkness that confronts us throughout our mortal life. If that light is obstructed – it can never be extinguished – we wander in a trackless waste devoid of purpose and consummated in futility. We read in the prologue of the fourth Gospel, 'All that came to be was alive with his life, and that life was the light of men. The light shines on in the dark, and the darkness has never mastered it' (John 1:4–5). The light of God is deeply implanted in the spirit of the soul, and the purpose and end of mortal life is to let that light pervade the whole personality, so that the occluding clouds of sinful desire are dissipated and finally transfigured into a warm glow of concern for the whole creation. This caring commences with our fellow men and extends ultimately to embrace the simplest form of life, even the most elementary particles of matter. God sent numerous religious teachers into the world at various times to enlighten their fellow men about the abundant life, which is ruined by the accumulated psychic burden of evil actions extending from the past. The way to deal with this is one of transmutation by perfect love, as was shown fully in the life of his Son, Jesus Christ. This is our vision also of the life that is perfect in quality: it is the way and the truth that alone show us God as Father, who loved the world so much that he gave his only Son that everyone who has faith in him may not die but have eternal life (John 3:16).

The man with one-pointed vision, the two eyes focused on a single point at a time, is symbolic of the person who has consecrated himself, his soul and body, to the service of his fellow creatures. When that service is dedicated to God's honour and glory, that person is a sacrament of the risen man in Christ. Now indeed the life he lives is more than merely his own life, but is also the life that Christ lives in him. In this respect, when we consider the implications of this insight of St Paul in Galatians 2:19, it is important to understand that our personal life is not summarily disrupted by the invasion of Christ into it, so that he forthwith takes it over for higher service. It is to be seen much more as an enrichment of our lives by the invitation of Christ to enter into our private home and bless its contents. He stands outside the gate of the soul, knocking to enter but waiting patiently to be admitted to what is, in effect, his own true domain. Though he is the true centre of the soul, the spirit – the life that is the light of man – until he is acknowledged with the totality of the personality, he remains outside our sanctuary. In this respect the saying of St James to the effect that even if a man keeps the whole Law apart from one single point, he is guilty of breaking it all (James 2:10), finds its positive application: until every aspect of ourself acknowledges Christ and lives according to that recognition, we fail to accept the full Christ into our lives, even though we may affirm his teachings with our mind and enter into his ministry with our emotions. The man whose spiritual eyes are sound and single in attention is filled with the light of Christ, and he is transfigured into his likeness, from splendour to splendour, such is the influence of the Lord who is Spirit (2 Cor. 3:18).

But, to return to Galatians 2:19 once more, the full life of Christ in the soul follows the experience of crucifixion with Christ. This means that all demands and expectations of the ego have to be put into their rightful place of subservience, if not total oblivion, before Christ can come into his own in the soul, now cleansed of the incubus of personal desire. This does not mean that desire in itself is reprehensible – Jesus himself said, 'How I have longed to eat this Passover with you before my death!' (Luke 22:15) – but that it becomes limiting when it is enclosed in personal ends devoid of a more communal concern. Jesus continues, in the passage quoted above, to prophesy that never again shall he eat the Passover until the time when it finds its fulfilment in the kingdom of God. At that time, which is the Parousia (the full coming of Christ in glory), the spiritual sight of all who participate in that meal, which commemorates the liberation of the children of Israel from Egyptian slavery, will be raised to envisage and enact the liberation of the whole created universe from the shackles of sinful self-regard to the freedom of self-expression sufficient to offer up everything to God in heaven.

This is the unobstructed vision that finds its end in a true healing, that one sees no longer 'puzzling reflections in a mirror, but face to face', with fullness of reality, as St Paul envisages in 1 Corinthians 13:12. This vision leads us on to the offering of our life to God's glory and our own resurrection. It is not a vision of happy repose and blissful comfort; on the contrary, it is one in which we have to experience death in the prospect of new life, a life as yet unknown but nevertheless fertile in promise of fulfilment. In the ministry of Ezekiel, the prophet both anticipates and participates in the sufferings of the exiled Jews – and therefore all Israel – by his own misfortunes. These are a sudden deprival of speech so that he is struck dumb for a considerable period of time, and the death of his beloved wife, whom he is forbidden to mourn openly. These are symbolic gestures of destruction of the whole nation, but the prophet does not merely carry out a mime, as in so many other rituals. Here his heart has to bleed in solidarity with a wicked people in their tragedy. But then comes the denouement: the promise of a regenerated nation portrayed by the marvellous vision of the valley full of bones that are resurrected to the stature of an immense living army. 'Prophesy, therefore, and say to them, These are the words of the Lord God: O my people, I will open your graves and bring you up from them, and restore you to the land of Israel. You shall know that I am the Lord when I open your graves and bring you up from them, O my people' (Ezek. 37:12–13). As the people revive, so does Ezekiel's speech return, and his prophecy ends on a triumphant note of the restored theocracy that is to herald a reformed Judaism, a Judaism inherited and fulfilled by Jesus some six centuries after Ezekiel's own ministry.

The experience of unobstructed vision occurred also in the life of St Paul, a man with a single mind even in his youth. He was so jealous for God's glory as an ardent Pharisee that he moved heaven and earth against the early Christian groups. He acquiesced in the stoning of Stephen as a dangerous force of subversion of the true faith, but during this whole period the Holy Spirit was working an inner revolution in his soul. When he was on the Damascus road, hot in pursuit of the Christians in that city, he was suddenly struck blind. The one-pointed vision of the past was not merely dimmed, it was completely obliterated. Now he laboured in complete darkness, in a cloud of absolute unknowing, as the risen Christ revealed himself and showed the former persecutor what he had to do with the remainder of his life. He was the one to be sent, the apostle, to the gentiles to bring them into a new relationship with God as revealed in Christ. Before Paul's spiritual vision could be cleared and redirected, his physical sight had to be temporarily dimmed so that he could experience the helplessness of a little child once more and receive healing at the hands of the disciple Ananias three days later. We remember once more the words of Christ in respect of the man born blind whom he had healed, 'It is for judgement that I have come into this world – to give sight to the sightless and to make blind those who see' (John 9:39–41). In the instance of St Paul the second action had to take precedence, for only in the darkness of complete incomprehension could his proud intellect and intolerant heart turn like a child to a new revelation of God. This revelation did not so much supplant his previous understanding of divine reality as bring it to a universal fulfilment. This fulfilment, this summing up of the Law as he was later to affirm, was based on the principle of love (Rom. 13:10), a particular quality that Paul was slowly to acquire in the course of his acquaintanceship with the risen Christ and the sufferings he was to endure in his service to him. Vision brings us all to a confrontation with what is eternal in each passing moment so that we can at last begin to devote our energies to the things that outlast the sensations of that moment.

Jesus says, 'You must work, not for this perishable food, but for the food that lasts, the food of eternal life' (John 6:27). This food, the Gospel goes on to explain, is given by Christ, upon whom God the Father has set his seal of authority. This seal is the Holy Spirit, who works the miracles that Jesus performs. What one sees with one's inner eye as a direct vision of the work ahead of one is articulated inwardly and interpreted by the inner ear as one's vocation. God calls each of us to some special work for the coming of his kingdom on earth. This does not mean that we all are called to some ministry, one which will direct us away from our mundane concerns into the arena of pure spiritual discipleship. It means rather that we have work to do here and now in forwarding the purpose of Christ on earth. While we are about our daily business, whether at home or doing some more specialized work in the larger world, we have a constant opportunity to spread God's love among those with whom we toil day by day. As we carry out God's business faithfully – as Jesus was about his Father's business even when he disputed with the teachers at the Temple when he was only twelve years old (Luke 2:41–51) – so we lose concern for ourselves and are filled increasingly with the Holy Spirit. To repeat 2 Corinthians 3:18, 'Because for us there is no veil over the face, we all reflect as in a mirror the splendour of the Lord; thus we are transfigured into his likeness, from splendour to splendour; such is the influence of the Lord who is Spirit'. The vision complemented by the inner call brings us to a full confrontation with the Holy Spirit, and our healing is now accelerated and consummated in God himself.

Each apparently menial task now assumes something of timeless heroism in the face of the uncomprehending darkness and blank apathy of those around us. Though they have eyes, they do not see; though they have ears, they do not hear – any more than did we before our inner vision was cleared and the inner voice became audible to us. The idols that the Prophets of Israel condemned so frequently also had the outer appurtenances that passed for sensory organs but lacked the living means to discern any stimulus. Man in his unredeemed state bears too close a resemblance to idols of wood and stone for any of us to be sanguine about his future. When, however, he is touched by the Spirit of God in a healing relationship, his outer organs of perception are not merely freed to do their proper work, but are also directed inwardly so that the spiritual content of their vision may be accepted, reflected upon and used constructively for the sake of the world. The call of God is to glorify him in whatever work we are doing amongst our brothers, so that the labour and its fulfilment may be a sacrament, leading us forward and inward to Christ himself. Jesus is conventionally portrayed as a carpenter who worked in Joseph's shop. I personally like to feel that he never lost contact with his trade even during the final period of his ministry among his brethren. Whatever he touched, he glorified. So too whatever is handled by a person imbued with the divine vision is consecrated to God's glory and the benefit of those who use it. The light of God transfigures material substance to spiritual essence, and all who partake of it are lifted up to God; it becomes a healing sacrament.

When Jesus performed his three resurrection miracles – the raising of Jairus' daughter, the widow of Nain's son, and Lazarus – he brought all three from death's shadow to a fresh vision of life, so that we may be sure the remainder of their days on earth were devoted to the things of eternity in a way that would previously have been inconceivable to them. We have all in due season to quit the physical body and enter into the life beyond death; this must surely have happened also to the three people whom Jesus raised. But their remaining life on earth was already an experience of resurrection. As St Paul puts it, 'When anyone is united to Christ, there is a new world; the old order has gone and a new order has already begun.' (2 Cor. 5:17). He goes on to say: 'From first to last this has been the work of God. He has reconciled us men to himself through Christ. ... God was in Christ reconciling the world to himself' (2 Cor. 5:18–19). Christ, in fact, by assuming men's sins, redeemed humanity from the bondage of sin, so that a new life of unobstructed vision was now possible, nothing less than the vision of God. When a person offers himself in openness of trust to God in Christ, he is cleansed of his past sinfulness, and the uncreated light of God can penetrate his whole being. This clears the portals of vision, so that now the person can discern and follow the light of God. This light, though of unfathomable radiance so that it blinds the mortal eye, as it did St Paul's eye in his experience on the road to Damascus, once it is accepted and accommodated by the soul, becomes a beacon of direction and a support of warm love. 'I am the light of the world. No follower of mine shall wander in the dark; he shall have the light of life' (John 8:12). The light is not only the medium of spiritual vision, it also opens the spiritual eyes to the perception of eternal truth, and so is the way, the truth and the very life of the one who knows Christ and lives by him. The unobstructed vision sees the truth that sets us free, and it informs the will so categorically that we start to move in the direction of that truth. The basis of the truth that sets us free is its property of leading us away from a selfish, sinful mode of existence to a knowledge of the eternal life in God. In other words, when the truth of Christ directs a person, he ceases to live a narrowly personal, acquisitive life, but instead enters a transpersonal mode of existence in which he lives for his neighbour's good also. The neighbour, as the Parable of the Good Samaritan tells us, is anyone in his proximity at any time and in any place. This was the life Jesus lived, and he has not inappropriately been called 'the man for others'.

Jesus' teaching about the life of vision, the transpersonal life, is direct and in harmony with the great mystics of all ages and traditions.

> Anyone who wishes to be a follower of mine must leave self behind; he must take up his cross and come with me. Whoever cares for his own safety is lost; but if a man will let himself be lost for my sake and for the Gospel, that man is safe. What does a man gain by winning the whole world at the cost of his true self? What can he give to buy that self back? (Mark 8:34–7)

It is of interest that six to eight days after giving this teaching, Jesus was transfigured in the sight of Peter, James and John. It was the vision of the three chosen disciples that was cleared and intensified by this event; for Jesus, who had always lived on this level of intimacy with the Father and love for his brethren, it was a presage of the resurrection later to follow. When one's vision has widened sufficiently to see one's neighbour as oneself, one has passed from the narrowly private personal existence we all guard so intensely to the transpersonal life in which the stranger is also a member of one's family. And that stranger then shows himself as the risen Lord, as he did to the travellers on the Emmaus road.

The measure of a truly spiritual healing is the steady transformation of the person's character so that he ceases to live for himself alone, but gives himself ever more unreservedly to others. His vision of fulfilment is no longer limited by the desire for personal gain. Instead the desire is for all people to gain a knowledge of God, in whom alone there is eternal life. As a person is healed spiritually, so he gives healing to others that in the end the whole world may be transfigured from dross to spiritual radiance. When Elisha prayed that his disciple – who was alarmed at the size of the enemy force surrounding them – might have his eyes opened so that he could see the angelic powers supporting them against their foes (2 Kings 6:17), he was anticipating the time when there would be such a general raising of consciousness amongst people that the invisible might be made fully visible. But spiritual vision is even more glorious than this enhanced psychic awareness; it articulates hope in the midst of desolation, and it energizes the faith that is a prerequisite for all fresh attempts in the future. It sees victory in apparent defeat, and it reckons that all things work together for good for those who love God (Rom. 8:28). That vision can never be obliterated, for it comes from God himself; it was the vision, already mentioned, of Ezekiel in the valley of bones that were resurrected to the strength of an immense living army. This vision can sustain us and empower our faith even during periods of terrible suffering and attrition.

A person is unlikely to relapse into past selfish ways of thought so long as his mind is imbued with the vision of progress, of growth, and ultimately of God himself. As St Paul writes in 2 Corinthians 4:16: 'No wonder we do not lose heart! Though our outward humanity is in decay, yet day by day we are inwardly renewed.' This inner renewal is effected by a fresh vision of the immortal splendour of God even when the earthly frame ages and perishes. 'Meanwhile our eyes are fixed, not on the things that are seen, but on the things that are unseen: for what is seen passes away; what is unseen is eternal' (2 Cor. 4:18). The unseen reality is sensed by the soul even in an unregenerate person, but as he is delivered from the slavery of his lower nature by the acceptance of Christ's unconditional love, so the doors of his inner perception are opened and widened. Then at last what he had vaguely felt in his depths now becomes a living reality. And the proof that the vision is real and not merely a comforting illusion is found in trusting it and following its illuminated path. It leads one to a full actualization of one's personality so that for the first time in one's life one can really see where one is going and co-operate joyfully with the process. The path is towards sharing in the very being of God (2 Peter 1:4) by entering 'mature manhood, measured by nothing less than the full stature of Christ' (Eph. 4:13). The full humanity is not merely individualistic, it involves the whole body of believers who will in due season include all humankind, indeed all creation. But it starts with the person who has passed from the death of purposelessness to the new life of hope revealed by the unfading vision of God's love.

And so it comes about that the congenitally blind man whom Jesus healed is a sacrament of the soul newly entered into divine knowledge where spiritual vision matches the gift of physical sight. While the intellectual giants may remain as spiritually blind in their conceit as ever, the humble soul who receives the gift of God's grace with the eagerness of a little child attains the vision of eternity. Indeed, it was well written, in Isaiah 11:6–9, that a little child will lead all the reconciled animals to the heavenly peace of the second Eden when the Messiah will have entered into his glory.

6

Deliverance from Evil

So they came to the other side of the lake, into the country
of the Gerasenes. As he stepped ashore, a man possessed
by an unclean spirit came up to him from among the
tombs where he had his dwelling. He could no longer be
controlled; even chains were useless; he had often been
fettered and chained up, but he had snapped the chains
and broken the fetters. No one was strong enough to master
him. And so, unceasingly, day and night, he would cry
aloud among the tombs and on the hill-sides and cut
himself with stones. When he saw Jesus in the distance, he
ran and flung himself down before him, shouting loudly,
'What do you want with me, Jesus, son of the Most High
God? In God's name do not torment me.' (For Jesus was
already saying to him, 'Out, unclean spirit, come out of
this man!') Jesus asked him, 'What is your name?' 'My
name is Legion,' he said, 'there are so many of us.' And
he begged hard that Jesus would not send them out of the
country. Now there happened to be a large herd of pigs
feeding on the hill-side, and the spirits begged him, 'Send
us among the pigs and let us go into them.' He gave them
leave; and the unclean spirits came out and went into the
pigs; and the herd, of about two thousand, rushed over the
edge into the lake and were drowned. (Mark 5:1–13)

The vision of the mind is often fitfully obstructed by thoughts and images projected from its unconscious depths. These are like wayward clouds that intercept the constant rays of the sun and cast their shadow on the ground. How frequently is an attempt at pure contemplation in the silence of God subverted by the emotional intrusion of ill-digested memories that impinge themselves upon the mind and will not be dislodged! How often also is the attention we ought to be giving to another person disrupted by material from the unconscious that brings with it a distasteful odour of past reminiscence! This casts its shadow on the present moment and robs the conversation of its tranquil intensity. The mind is all too often a seething cauldron of unhealed memories of past failure that blight our present equanimity and condemn us to future inadequacy, if not complete impotence. The names of the legion of hosts that possess the unquiet mind are anxiety, fear, envy, resentment, anger, lust, pride, suspicion and ill-will. We have inherited them as part of the conditioning we underwent during the formative years of our upbringing, and their number is steadily increased by the sordid life we live and our unsatisfactory relationships with other people.

Every action brings its corresponding reaction. The law of relationships is very plain. 'Pass no judgement, and you will not be judged. For as you judge others so you will yourselves be judged, and whatever measure you deal out to others will be dealt back to you' (Mat. 7:1–2). St Paul expands on this theme of retribution, 'Make no mistake about this: God is not to be fooled; a man reaps what he sows. If he sows seed in the field of his lower nature, he will reap from it a harvest of corruption, but if he sows in the field of the Spirit, the Spirit will bring him a harvest of eternal life' (Gal. 6:7–8). The importance of confessing our sins in order to obtain free forgiveness from God has already been discussed; there can be no permanent healing while the mind is clouded by existential guilt, by which I mean a feeling of guilt for a sin that has been deliberately committed and whose repercussions disturb the psychic atmosphere. But the mind is a seething mass of conflicting emotions. We have both sinned and been sinned against. Much sin is the result of the resentment and distrust that have arisen inside ourselves from injustice we have suffered and betrayal we have undergone at the hands of those whom we had innocently trusted. The emotional contortions of a darkened mind cannot be easily fathomed, let alone healed. Confession cannot become meaningful until the mental contents have been sorted out and analysed with clear, rational discernment.

It is from this cesspit of unassimilated emotional debris that the evil actions of men emanate. What we ourselves have failed to obtain we tend to covet in others. What we lack we envy in our neighbour. What lies beyond our reach we will strive to demolish in someone more gifted than ourselves, in the process seeking to destroy, if not his life, then at least his reputation. There is, I believe, a radical destructive tendency in human nature which, if released, could reduce the whole world to chaos, undoing God's own creative act of the beginning of time. This dark, demonic force shows itself disconcertingly when we gloat over the fall of the righteous and speak evil of those whom the world esteems. The naked pleasure that many of the spectators at Calvary showed as Jesus suffered his final humiliation on the cross is matched throughout all ages by the glee with which minority groups have been persecuted because of their racial origin, religious belief or style of life. If this persecution can be carried out in the name of God or common morality, the satisfaction is all the greater. It is indeed an enormous relief to project one's own inner disorder on to a helpless victim, who becomes a scapegoat. But the hatred so generated will pursue its own malign momentum in the collective psychic atmosphere long after its victim has been disposed of and destroyed.

The origin of evil is itself something of an enigma. Some believe it is essentially an absence of goodness, and that it has no substantive existence of its own. The barbarity of man to his fellows, epitomized in the unsurpassed cruelty of the concentration camps of our own century, suggests that there is more to evil than a mere absence of goodness; it seems to have its own powerful identity even if its end is negative. Others attribute evil to ignorance, often rather glibly; the calculated tortures that punctuate not a few personal relationships as well as the prison camps already alluded to, point not so much to ignorance as to the unqualified enjoyment some warped personalities derive from hurting their fellow creatures. In the perversion of sadism this enjoyment has strong sexual overtones. The evil that has been inflicted on one group will very probably be visited later by them on others weaker than they, as they strive for the protection that power appears to provide. This vicious circle will continue until human consciousness undergoes a radical change in perspective; thus deliverance from the power of evil is a vital part of the ministry of healing, but is often not confronted directly in this light.

It would seem that evil has a collective origin, and arises from an abuse of the free will God has bestowed on his rational creatures. Its ultimate origin may indeed stem from ignorance – as symbolized in the story of the Fall, where Adam and Eve chose the knowledge of good and evil on a separative, acquisitive human level, rather than eternal life in God, from whom all wisdom comes. When we set ourselves up privately apart from others, rivalry and hostility are inevitable by-products of our individualistic endeavours until we grasp the truth that our own well-being depends on that of the society around us, and that success on a separative level is ephemeral and illusory. It is in giving our unique contribution to the whole that we cease to be a small, separate unit and become instead a vital part of the community. And then life in eternity opens up its welcome embrace even to us, the least of mortals. But once we have entered on the separative path, the consequences of our actions mount up within us and are discharged into the psychic atmosphere in which we live our inner life and communicate most intimately with those around us. The statement sometimes made that thoughts are things, though facile, has a real truth behind it. Our perverse inclinations poison the atmosphere around us, and if unredeemed can have an adverse effect on those who follow us on the path of life. On occasions these thought processes can assume a tangible form, and as such may be sensed by those who are sensitive psychically. These apparitions are, however, merely the tip of an iceberg of psychic debris that infests the inner world of aspiration, thought and relationships in which we live most vibrantly and from which the ultimate scale of values is derived. It is as a person thinks in the depths of his being, the soul, that marks his character and his relationships with others.

Evil cannot be spirited away by shallow rationalization. Each generation may give it a new name according to a current vogue in psychological or sociological thought, but in the end the evil tendency has to be isolated, exorcised and then redeemed. There are in this respect two practical aspects of evil; that which emanates directly from a person as the result of a moral disorder within him, and that which infests society as a whole, from which it may be concentrated on especially vulnerable people. This vulnerability depends on the person's innate psychic constitution and his family and cultural background. The two work closely together: even a very psychically sensitive person is unlikely to be the receptacle of evil forces so long as he lives an upright, morally aspiring life. In this respect membership of a worshipping community, one whose inner sight is directed to the Deity however he may be known, is of great protective value. In the end the moral law is obeyed, not by the fear of retribution in the event of one's being caught and unmasked by the stern, rather impersonal forces of justice in a community, but by a deeper love for all creation. St Paul spoke truly when he said that the whole law is summed up by love (Rom. 13:10); it is fulfilled in loving concern to all our neighbours. Indeed, the deliverance of a person from evil impulses –. whether these stem from within him or have invaded him from without – is essentially a labour of love, an attitude that sees the other person as infinitely valuable and is prepared to give up everything for him.

Love is very different from sentimental effusiveness in which moral judgement is suspended so that the most evil actions are condoned, perhaps after being conveniently explained in terms of background and heredity. Love is a direct, fearless confrontation with the other person in which the totality of his inner life is accepted and exchanged in trust. Then comes the judgement, and this is passed by the person himself, perhaps acting in collaboration with the minister of healing. When Jesus attended the revelries of the lower strata of his society, he was performing a supreme healing act. It is probable that even he did not see it in this light, for if he had been too solicitous about the moral well-being of the revellers, an unpleasant aura of sanctimony would have intruded itself to the detriment of a perfect relationship between himself and the others. A perfect relationship is gauged by its transparency, that nothing need be hidden and the heart is completely open. In the open heart God shows himself even in the person of a very great sinner. The tragedy of the sinner is that his habitual attitude of selfishness obstructs the living God within, whereas those who aspire to a nobler way of life are increasingly open to the divine source inside themselves.

The healing Jesus performed in his social engagements was simply that of giving his essence to all who would receive it. Though he knew the baseness of the life of a prostitute, a drunkard or a dishonest tax-gatherer, he did not associate the trade or the weakness with the person he was then confronting. What he saw was a child of his Father, one who had fallen lamentably from his high calling as a son fashioned in the divine image, but one who nevertheless was a brother. To be with Jesus was to receive love, a love that penetrated to the depths of the personality and called the person once more to fulfil the divine imperative within him. This imperative is always the same: a limitless goodness comparable with that of our heavenly Father (Mat. 5:48). This goodness is made manifest in unconditional love, as the preceding sentences of the Sermon on the Mount make quite clear. It was the virtuous who often felt most threatened by Christ, because outer moral rectitude can be devoid of a deeper compassion for the pariahs of society. A morality without love soon deteriorates into a zeal for condemnation and persecution; indeed, evil flourishes best in such a milieu because it can hide behind the bastions of propriety and religion, even the name of the Deity.

Evil tendencies have therefore to be uncovered, preferably by the loving insight of the one who ministers healing; it is here that counselling and healing converge into the simple point of transfiguration. Once the evil has been acknowledged it should be given to God in prayer; the invoked presence of Jesus in the imagination can be of great help in this transaction to those who are committed Christians, but a great deal depends on the person's temperament. The minister of healing should share in the burden with the sinner, helping to relieve him of the terrible incubus of inner darkness in silent contemplation. This work of intimate psychic support is the crown of the healing process, and it may be consummated by the laying-on of hands as a sacramental gesture of the downpouring of the Holy Spirit on the personality now disembarrassed of its evil tendency. At this stage a confession is valuable; the confessor need not be a priest, but he must be a person of love and moral stature capable of bearing the substance confessed and interceding with God on the sinner's behalf. We have already considered St James' advice in respect of the sick, of confessing our sins to one another, praying for one another and expecting healing (Jas. 5:16). In all this work scrupulous reticence is essential, comparable with the trust invested in a doctor who may be called on to hear the deepest secrets of a patient's life. It follows that no one should enter the healing ministry until he has attained that degree of discretion not to become entangled in the private life of the person he is serving and that moral excellence not to take advantage of anyone who puts himself under his care.

Love is quiet and effective in its embracing, healing activity. It cannot force itself on the object of its concern; it can only wait to be summoned, since it does not invade the personality or wear down the will of the one in need of help. When a person steadfastly refuses to confront the corruption within him or else simply rationalizes it away in terms of his past background, he will remain in bondage to it. So long as one clings voluntarily to a past attitude one remains subject to all its limitations and constraints. Christ himself cannot act against a person's will; he can only stand patiently and wait to be called. But when he is called, he immediately takes control of the situation and will not relinquish it until complete healing has been attained. This means that love is strong and directive; it will never let go even if it has to force the beloved to see the truth of the situation. The relationship between God and the Jews is a perfect demonstration of this truth in the whole sequence of the Old Testament. On a more personal, universal level Christ continues this work in the new dispensation. This forcing of the beloved to face the reality of his sinfulness and the consequences that have flowed from it in terms of ruined opportunities, broken relationships and shattered health is of the essence of deliverance from personal evil. Relationships are an especially valuable gauge of one's inner life: the two attitudes that are especially important in destroying them are insensitivity and treachery. There can be no inner healing so long as either of these prevail; insensitivity shields us from the living power of the Holy Spirit, while treachery separates us from the joyous community of life that is brought together by the Holy Spirit.

There is, however, a more collective aspect of evil that has already been mentioned. Evil inclinations pollute the psychic atmosphere, and sometimes they are attached to discarnate entities on the other side of death, which is in all probability, on the lower levels, much like our present life in general tone. This is where the ministry of deliverance becomes an important aspect of the work of healing. In Jesus' time this ministry was accepted without question, but nowadays the tendency is to attribute all perverse inclinations to the person himself and dismiss as illusory any source of interference outside the personal psyche that does not reach it in a rational or sensory way. On the whole this tendency is to be welcomed, as it dispenses with much thought process that smacks of primitive superstition. Nevertheless, there are occasions when an outside influence does appear to be at work in causing internal havoc in a person already subject to mental or emotional disturbance, and the disposal of this mischievous influence can lighten the burden of the afflicted one considerably. The work of sensing such an influence is specialized, being the prerogative of a person with the gift of discernment of spirits. Some people have this psychic sensitivity as a natural endowment, whereas others appear to acquire it as they grow in spiritual maturity. The second way is preferable, because the discernment develops as a gift of spiritual grace, an acquisition on the rungs of the spiritual ladder. But the naturally gifted psychic is not to be discouraged, let alone discountenanced. Many people with a natural healing gift come into this category. What is required in such an innately

sensitive person is a life of spiritual aspiration with the three
beacons of prayer, worship in a believing community and
service to the world outside, leading him on to a full encounter
with God and with himself. If these prerequisites of the spiritual life are ignored or taken lightly, the gift may well become
contaminated by the acquisitiveness of the personal ego and
the personality itself infested by dark demonic powers emanating from the psychic realm.

The question of what St Paul calls 'our fight, which is not
against human foes, but against cosmic powers, against the
authorities and potentates of this dark world, against the
superhuman forces of evil in the heavens' (Eph. 6:12), always
evokes strong feelings. The humanistic type of religionist
tends to scoff at the concept of powers of evil in realms beyond
human experience; he usually also has considerable difficulty
in believing in life after death of the physical body. The
enthusiastic exorcist, on the other hand, tends to see all
difficulties and disappointments as the fruit of the attack of
dark forces on the powers of light. The devil, however we
may portray him – and he is a convenient symbol at the very
least for the forces of darkness in and around us that would
lead to general destruction if given free rein – has a cosmic
power, but in the end all things work together for good for
those who love God (Rom. 8:28). The risen man in Christ
learns the supreme art of loving his enemies and praying for
his persecutors (Mat. 5:44). This is no permissive tolerance
but a warm compassion that sees all things potentially
redeemed by the love of Christ and renewed by the power of
the Holy Spirit. The ancient Jewish understanding that God
is the master of good and evil should always be borne in
mind: 'I am the Lord, there is no other; I make the light, I
create darkness, author alike of prosperity and trouble' (Isa.
45:7). The downpouring of darkness and trouble on the world
is no doubt the result of secondary causes related to the
ignorance and perverted will of the creature, whether angelic,
human or of some other order, but God is in ultimate control
and can be called on for help by the action of prayer. This
essential spiritual practice re-aligns the will, so that we cease
to do evil and start to do good, as the prophets of old were
constantly exhorting the Jews.

St Paul says, 'Adapt yourselves no longer to the pattern of this present world, but let your minds be remade and your whole nature thus transformed. Then you will be able to discern the will of God, and to know what is good, acceptable and perfect' (Rom. 12:2). This process of remaking of the mind is effected by the humility of self-awareness and the ardent aspiration of rapt prayer. And then the gift of discernment is made manifest and sharpened to knife-edge discrimination. As one grows in spiritual light, so the other person becomes as close to one as one's own soul; indeed, the love of neighbour as of self reaches its final fulfilment – not as a fleeting rapture, but as a constant awareness. The growth into the knowledge of God's love brings us to the heart of all suffering creation. As we share in Christ's persistent agony – until the end of the world of separation – so we bring his compassion and light to all who suffer and are disfigured in body, mind and soul.

In this way the sinner is loved as oneself and the sin banished to the world beyond our knowing where God's healing grace may be bestowed even on that perverted quality. In the ministry of deliverance the invading entity is called out in the name of God the Father, the Son and the Holy Spirit. But it is not simply left to perish – if indeed this were possible – in the outer darkness. It is directed in the name of love and by the power of the uncreated light of God to enter that place in the world beyond death that God has prepared for it in his infinite caring. The story of the pigs into which the evil spirits were let loose, which prefixed this chapter, and their tumultuous rush into the lake where they were drowned is surely only the outer manifestation of an awesome, indeed terrible, event. In the depths into which pigs and spirits were alike directed one may be sure that the love of God was not in abeyance. As we read in Psalm 139:8, 'If I climb up to heaven, thou art there; if I make my bed in Sheol, again I find thee.' God's omnipresence is the surety of our salvation once we have had the faith and wisdom to call upon him in prayer. In an act of deliverance the departing entities must be directed to God's love, and the person (or place) now cleansed must be blessed, while the power of the Holy Spirit is called upon to fill him (or it) with new life.

Furthermore, the prayer of a loving group should continue unabated for some days after the deliverance. It is much easier to dislodge a focus of evil than to replace it with a presence of peace and love. The story of the entity who returns with seven more of its own kind, even worse than itself, which we have already considered, must never be far from the thoughts of anyone involved in the work of deliverance. The person now delivered must be instructed in the life of prayer, scripture-reading and worship in a devout community. He must also devote time to the service of those less fortunate than himself. These are the ways in which reinfestation is prevented, and they are clearly an integral part of the full ministry of healing.

It is usual to consider healing as something given to an afflicted person from outside, especially through the agency of one who ministers to him. But in fact this is merely the initial phase. The end of such preliminary healing is to awaken and strengthen the inner healing power of the person himself. The *vis medicatrix naturae* that infuses the living body has its subtler and more potent counterparts in the realms of the mind and the soul. Only when these too are activated can the person start to lead a new life of release from past destructive attitudes and enter into joyful participation in the present moment. The risen life, which we at least glimpse even now, is one of open receptivity to the glory of the present moment, which is our immediate taste of eternity. This open receptivity is blocked by evil, separative impulses within us that shut out the rays of God's love from the soul within. Therefore a fundamental aspect of healing work is the remaking of the mind and a transformation of the whole nature, to quote Romans 12:2 once more. Certainly the skills of psychotherapy can play an important part in this process, but before these can be fully effective there must be a firm confrontation of the forces of evil, both personal and communal. Only when these have been disposed of can the deeper healing of the mind be initiated.

It should finally be stated categorically that the possibility of evil infestation of the personality by outside forces does not annul the principle of personal responsibility. It is the disturbed person who is most liable to such invasion by outside forces, and until his own house is put in order once more, he will be subject to recurrent harassment from without. As Jesus says in respect of the return of the Master at the end of time, 'Even if it is the middle of the night or before dawn when he comes, happy are they if he finds them alert. And remember, if the householder had known what time the burglar was coming, he would not have let his house be broken into' (Luke 12:38–39). If this applies to the believer at the Second Coming of the Lord, it is even more immediately pertinent to the invasion of a torpid, complacent personality by the forces of evil. These fester at the root of the unredeemed ego, and lurk menacingly in the defiled psychic atmosphere from which we all derive our daily emotional sustenance.

The people whom Jesus delivered from the power of evil – whether of an inner disposition or of an outer infestation – are the sacraments of a new order of men with unclouded minds and radiant vision. They reveal the 'right mindfulness' so stressed by the Buddha some six hundred years before Christ's advent. In fact, one can work with one-pointed application to the moment in hand only when one's mind is cleansed of evil encumbrances. The grace of God initiates this healing work once the will to be changed has been activated. And then the life of 'meditation in action' proceeds. At first it may be fitful and disturbed, but as one grows in spiritual proficiency and humility, so it remains with one to become a constant blessing. This is the path of ministering healing to a world so distraught with trivialities that it is seldom aware of the undying love of God.

7

The Sacraments in Healing

In truth, in very truth I tell you, unless you eat the flesh of the Son of Man and drink his blood you have no life in you. Whoever eats my flesh and drinks my blood possesses eternal life, and I will raise him up on the last day. My flesh is real food; my blood is real drink. Whoever eats my flesh and drinks my blood dwells continually in me and I dwell in him. As the living Father sent me, and I live because of the Father, so he who eats me shall live because of me. This is the bread which came down from heaven; and it is not like the bread which our fathers ate: they are dead, but whoever eats this bread shall live for ever.

(John 6:53–8)

Every object, indeed every event in our lives, is potentially a sacrament. It is an outward sign and portent of a spiritual reality, for, as Psalm 24 tells us, 'The earth is the Lord's and all that is in it, the world and those who dwell therein'. The creation, from the minutest crystal to the most majestic mountain peak, the simplest unicellular organism to man at his most godlike, is fully subject to the divine creative will, and is sustained and loved by God. We remember in this context Dame Julian of Norwich and her exquisite revelation:

Also in this he shewed me a little thing, the quantity of an hazel-nut in the palm of my hand; and it was as round as a ball. I looked thereupon with eye of my understanding, and thought: What may this be? And it was answered generally thus: It is all that is made. I marvelled how it might last, for methought it might suddenly have fallen to naught for littleness. And I was answered in my understanding: It lastest and shall ever last for that God loveth it. And so All-thing hath the Being by the love of God. In this Little Thing I saw three properties. The first is that God made it, the second that God loveth it, the third that God keepeth it. (*Revelations of Divine Love*, chapter 5)

The divine essence is not foreign to the smallest creature, for the Holy Spirit, the Lord and giver of all life, infuses and sustains the entire universe. In this respect it is man's supreme privilege to know the Holy Spirit as a divine presence within his own soul and to co-operate with him in the resurrection of the world. What a marvellous creature the human being is in truth, bringing into creative union the physical and the spiritual by way of the psychical! He is God's collaborator in our world, when he works according to the priesthood bestowed on him. He acts perpetually as intercessor for the world to God, as did Moses on behalf of the recalcitrant Israelites or Jesus for those who had participated in his crucifixion. 'Father, forgive them; they do not know what they are doing' (Luke 23:34).

This statement of Christ on the cross incriminates ignorance as the basic cause of much, if not all, evil. It is the antithesis of the sacramental universe. The intrinsic holiness of all matter, which we have already noted, depends on the human touch for its sanctity to be made manifest in the world. It is here that the priesthood of man, of the entire human stock, finds its apogee. Whatever is handled and used with reverence and love in the name of God is consecrated to his use and becomes an object of blessing. Without in any way ceasing to be itself with its own intrinsic properties, it also finds its ultimate meaning in the realm of eternity. Therefore any work done in devotion to God, from whom all life and healing proceed, and in love to our fellow creatures carries with it a divine blessing. It blesses alike the one who gives and the one who receives. In between the two, lies God the

Holy Spirit. It follows that no work is intrinsically menial or noble: its quality depends on the attitude and awareness of the person who performs it. The ablution of a latrine or the cleaning of soiled bedclothes can be as close to God's service as is the act of consecration of the elements of the Eucharist by a priest or the composition of a great work by an inspired artist. The food that a housewife prepares in love for those she serves is no mean presage of the eternal food God gives unceasingly of himself for our sustenance and healing.

The holiness of matter was proclaimed finally and definitively when the Word became fully flesh and dwelt among us, and we saw his glory, such glory as befits the Father's only Son, full of grace and truth (John 1:14). That flesh was ultimately, after it had suffered the ignominy of betrayal, the pain of physical torture and the agony of psychic darkness, to be resurrected to full spiritual reality. It was to share in the very being of God as a presage of the time when matter itself will no longer be subject to the deterioration inherent in mortality and find instead its true place in the eternal life of God. And even now any physical object that is handled in love and blessed in the name of the Almighty, retains the benediction and can transfer the love to the person who receives it. On the level of personal relationships a gift can bring gladness to the heart out of all proportion to its intrinsic value if it is given in love. On the spiritual level the things of our world can proclaim the nature of their Creator when they are blessed in his name. While never ceasing to retain their own identity, they at the same time are lifted above the rut of common usage to participate in the very nature of eternal life. Thus when even two or three have met together in the name of Christ, he is there among them (Mat. 18:20). His presence blesses them and fulfils the prayers they utter.

When Adam and Eve reject the invitation to enjoy the perpetual fellowship of God by choosing wilfully to investigate the knowledge of good and evil on a purely rational level – a symbolic exaltation of themselves above the divine providence, which is now relegated to the background of their thoughts – they exclude themselves from paradise, the garden of Eden in the creation story. God says to Adam that, because of his own and his wife's disobedience, the very ground is accursed on their account. With labour alone they will from henceforth win their food from it all the days of their life, and it will grow thorns and thistles, nothing but wild plants for them to eat. They will gain their bread by the sweat of their brows until they too rejoin the ground – from it they were taken and to it they will return as dust (Gen. 3:17–19). The sacrament of purifying labour – symbolized in the sweat of the brow – sets in motion the sanctification of man's selfish, predatory control over material life which is an inevitable fruit of a separative knowledge of good and evil. The good and evil that concerns unredeemed man has a purely selfish application: that which benefits him materially is identified as his good, while that which stands in his way is regarded as evil. In this very childish understanding of values, man's sight is limited by expediency in terms of time and egoism in terms of extent. The deeper understanding that ultimate good must include all creation, and that the present moment is a passing illusion when separated from its place in the whole of life is beyond the comprehension of the naked human intellect. The recurrent pain and disappointment, succeeded by the renewed hope embodied in physical labour, start the process of restoring the earth from the curse of corruption to the promise of resurrection.

The products of the earth can be epitomized in the bread of daily sustenance and the wine that restores the warmth of life after a day's heavy toil. In the totally unredeemed person's life these products of the earth are purely symbols of gluttony and debauchery: to eat and drink to one's physical satiety is the summation of purpose in life. St Paul would put it thus, 'If the dead are never raised to life, let us eat and drink, for tomorrow we die' (1 Cor. 15:32), as he quotes bitingly a popular maxim. As the person grows in love, so the bread and wine of common life are symbols of hospitality; they are given to refresh and restore the stranger on the rugged path of daily toil. Finally, when they are consecrated to God they become the very essence of life, for now they are the body and blood of Christ himself. Thus we read, 'Unless you eat the flesh of the Son of Man and drink his blood you can have no life in you. Whoever eats my flesh and drinks my blood possesses eternal life, and I will raise him up on the last day'

(John 6:53–54), words that prefixed this chapter. Jesus also tells us that the Spirit alone gives life, and that the flesh is of no avail (John 6:63). It is the Holy Spirit infusing the substance of the world that makes it holy; this holiness is made real by the action of the human being when he consecrates himself and all he uses to God's glory and the service of his fellow creatures. In the instance of the manna provided for the Israelites during their journey across the desert to the Promised Land, Jesus tells the Jews that it was not Moses who gave the heavenly bread, but God who gives of himself perpetually for the love he bears his creatures. Jesus says he is the bread of life and that only those who come to him will never be hungry and those who believe in him will thirst no more (John 6:32–5). The work of Jesus, therefore, is of a very different order of being from that of the magician or psychic miracle-worker who changes stones to bread. This, in fact, was one of Jesus' temptations while he was in the wilderness. Had he obliged the devil on this occasion by producing such a phenomenon, he would simply have exhibited his psychic proficiency, and in the end he might easily have enslaved all those who submitted themselves to him in the guise of a remarkable miracle worker. The final master in such a transaction is the devil himself. By contrast, the providence of Jesus in such a miracle as the multiplication of the loaves and fishes is one of perpetual self-giving to the multitudes, who are like hungry sheep without a caring shepherd. Their hunger is not merely physical but much more urgently spiritual. The sacraments of the Church remind us that Christ has given unceasingly of himself for the creation of all the material of the world, and when it is blessed in his name, he is there among all who are assembled as well as in the physical object itself, which then bears a blessing that both heals and restores.

And so it comes about that the Eucharist is the principal healing sacrament of the Church. But it also reminds us that all we eat and drink have a sacramental quality when they are prepared, handled and consumed in reverence and thanksgiving. In Ezekiel's vision of the miraculous spring that issues from the precincts of the Temple and becomes a wide, flowing river, the banks are lined with trees bearing fruit of life-renewing power (Ezek. 47:1–12). In the account of the New Jerusalem that concludes the Book of Revelation, this vision is broadened to attain cosmic dimensions: 'Then he showed me the river of the water of life, sparkling like crystal, flowing from the throne of God and of the Lamb down the middle of the city's street. On either side of the city stood a tree of life, which yields twelve crops of fruit, one for each month of the year; the leaves of the trees serve for the healing of the nations' (Rev. 22:1–2). In the consecrated world each living form becomes edible not only for physical sustenance but also for spiritual transformation.

The water of life starts as a cleansing material. When Jesus uses it to wash the feet of his disciples just before his own betrayal and death, he brings to that basic element of nature, so taken for granted, the qualities of humility, service and purification. When it is used in the sacrament of Holy Baptism, it is a symbol of death of the old personality and a resurrection of the soul into a new life, one indeed of intimate sharing of the life of Christ. 'Have you forgotten that when we were baptised into union with Christ Jesus we were baptised into his death? By baptism we were buried with him, and lay dead, in order that, as Christ was raised from the dead in the splendour of the Father, so also we might set our feet upon the new path of life' (Rom. 6:3–4). In the old dispensation, the sea has an evil connotation – it also symbolizes the unconscious mind – so that in the new heaven and earth there is no longer any sea (Rev. 21:1). It has been lifted up and spiritualized, when all who have passed through the barrier of mortal death have entered into the new life in God. Baptism is the initial healing sacrament; it brings the person symbolically through death and isolation into the community of all believers. The work is continued in the healing elements of the Eucharist, and is completed in all the elements of the world which we handle, use and eat. Consecrated water brings a blessing on psychically disturbed premises once the invading entity has been sent on its way for its own healing. In the healing of Naaman the Syrian by Elisha, the word of God works through the medium of the cleansing waters of the Jordan; they carry the blessing that removes the disfiguring skin disease from the army commander once he attains sufficient humility to immerse himself in the river seven times. The cleansing function of the water opens and illuminates the soul of Naaman so that he now acknowledges the one true God. Herein lies an even deeper healing, of which the restored surface is an outer sign.

The other great healing sacrament, Holy Unction, the anointing of the sick person with consecrated oil, stems from the use of oil in anointing the head of a guest as a gesture of hospitality (Ps. 23:5). Oil is at once enriching, lubricating and of a soothing nature. Mixed with various spices, the oil of the olive was used in the solemn act of anointing priests and kings in the time of the Old Testament (Exod. 30:22–33). The sacrament of anointing makes the king or priest a holy person, the anointed of God, the Messiah in the case of a king (or the Christ, as it is translated in Greek). But oil has also been used to anoint the sick; until recently the rite was employed almost exclusively for a dying person and was called extreme unction, but nowadays it is widely used for those who are ill. 'Is one of you ill? He should send for the elders of the congregation to pray over him and anoint him with oil in the name of the Lord. The prayer offered in faith will save the sick man, the Lord will raise him from his bed, and any sins he may have committed will be forgiven. Therefore confess your sins to one another, and pray for one another, and then you will be healed' (Jas. 5:14–16). In this succinct, though remarkably comprehensive, advice St James summarizes the essential aspects of spiritual healing: prayer, anointing and confession with absolution. When a person is anointed in the name of the Lord, the oil transmits the holy benediction and brings about an inward change in the one who receives it. But first there should be, if possible, a time for counselling that ends with a confession and absolution, followed by a period of prayer together, before the anointing is performed. In the instance of a desperately ill person this sequence must necessarily be severely curtailed.

In the beautifully evocative Psalm 133 the intimate love of fraternal communion is compared with the oil of consecration poured liberally over Aaron's head and running over his face and vestments. It blesses, not only the great high priest, but also all who are united in the priesthood as symbolized by

71

the vestments: it is the destiny of the children of Israel to become a nation of priests (Exod. 19:6). All human beings are meant ultimately to exercise the authority of priests before God in representing the natural world before him and elevating it for blessing before its final transfiguration. Oil mixed with costly spices was used by the woman who came to anoint Jesus' body just before his passion and death; it was her way of preparing him for burial (Mark 14:3–9). After the burial that same body was to be resurrected into full spiritual radiance; the oil too had played its humble part in the cosmic conflict ahead of the Master, his agony, death and final triumph. In a much diminished form all healing sacraments are to be seen in this light: even when they appear to fail in their immediate object of inducing a natural cure, they are preparing the victim for the next stage in his spiritual journey that ends in the vision of God.

In the sacramental approach to healing, a part of the minister's own body is added to the natural elements of the world. The elements of the Eucharist – the bread and the wine – are prepared by human hands from the time that the wheat is sown and reaped and the vine tended and harvested, up to the preparation of the final products: as we have seen, God decreed that man shall gain his bread by the sweat of his brow (Gen. 3:19). And then the Eucharist is prepared on the altar by the president, an act that culminates in the final consecration of the elements to be distributed. In some of Jesus' healing miracles he uses his own spittle as part of the sacrament: in the healing of the man born blind, for instance, Jesus spat on the ground and made a paste with the spittle, which he spread on the man's eyes. Then he ordered him to wash in the pool of Siloam. When the man had done this, he could see for the first time in his life (John 9:6–7). This episode bears a resemblance to the healing of Naaman's skin disease: the healing was initiated by the word of Elisha as communicated by his servant and completed by Naaman's sevenfold immersion in the waters of the Jordan. In the sacramental act of laying-on of hands the minister of healing gives of his very body to be used by the power of the Holy Spirit. In this respect the words of St Teresa of Avila are especially relevant: 'Remember, Christ has no body now on earth but yours, no hands but yours, no feet but yours. Yours are the eyes through which must look out Christ's compassion on the world. Yours are the feet with which he is to go about doing good. Yours are the hands with which he is to bless men now.'

Indeed, the physical body given in service is a mighty sacrament. Hands used to calm, comfort and restore a fellow creature who is bereft and terrified are involved as intimately in the work of healing as when they are employed in some conventionally religious act. The priest himself is a sacrament of Christ's universal presence when he pronounces the words of absolution. Many of us still unfortunately have an adverse attitude towards the body, due in large measure to the way mankind has abused it through neglect, gluttony and debauchery. The use of spittle offends our contemporary approach to hygiene, yet saliva is endowed with disinfectant properties. If our mouths were clean, the saliva would be fresh and healing in power; when our mouths are poorly cleansed, our breath soiled through smoking and alcohol, and our teeth rotten due to dietary indiscretion, then too does the spittle become offensive. Health is indivisible, permeating the entire personality from the soul to the body by way of the mind and the emotions. St Paul reminds us very forcibly that the body is a shrine of the indwelling Holy Spirit, and the Spirit is God's gift to us. Indeed we do not belong to ourselves, for we were bought (by Christ, who redeemed us from the slavery of sin) at a price. We should therefore honour God in our body (1 Cor. 6:19–20).

But in fact the whole world is a sacrament; it is we in our obtuse self-centredness who avert our gaze from the transcendent splendour around us that also shows us the way to a knowledge of God. Jean-Pierre de Caussade in his spiritual classic *Self-Abandonment to Divine Providence* speaks near the beginning of the first section, on the virtue of self-abandonment, of the sacrament of the present moment. He considers, as an example, the external life of the Blessed Virgin which was on the surface very simple and ordinary. She did and experienced much the same things as did other people in her state of life at that particular time. Outwardly the events of her life after the birth of Jesus were little different from those

73

which happen to everyone, but the interior invisible element that can be discerned by faith is nothing less than God himself performing these works. De Caussade sees in the bread of angels, the heavenly manna, the pearl of the Gospels, nothing but the sacrament of the present moment. God the Son is present in such lowly surroundings as the manger, the hay and the straw. Furthermore he was given not to the mighty but to the humble. 'The hungry he has satisfied with good things, the rich sent empty away' (Luke 1:53). God reveals himself to the humble in the humblest things, while the great of this world who never penetrate beneath the surface do not discover him even in great events.

The sacraments of the Church remind us of the holiness of all creation. God created them all and he saw that it was good, as the first chapter of the Genesis story puts it. The humbler creatures are given over to human dominion, and even the perverted will of the rational creature cannot entirely destroy the other forms of existence. It certainly defiles them, in so doing bringing suffering into the world, but the fruits of this very sinfulness are the means whereby the gradually enlightened will of man can begin to repair some of the damage he and his forebears have done. Once man returns to God in prayer, he can at last begin to heal the harmful effects of the past. Prayer makes possible the entry of the Holy Spirit as a conscious presence into the world of matter, which now can assume a sacramental form. When man is fully enlightened by the will of God – when his whole life is prayer – he will see the divine presence in each moment of time. The need for special sacraments will dissolve into the awareness of the sacramental nature of the world, and every moment will be glorified by the living God.

The greatest sacrament in the world of becoming is the Church, described as the mystical body of Christ, since the body of the risen Christ is to be the focus of worship in spirit and truth. In the final advent, symbolized as the New Jerusalem in the Book of Revelation, there is to be no concrete church any longer: 'I saw no temple in the city; for its temple was the sovereign Lord God and the Lamb' (Rev. 21:22). Then, as is prophesied, the Lord shall be one Lord and his name the one name (Zech. 14:9). In our present world the sacraments of the Church are of the greatest value in reminding us of the holiness of even the simplest products of the soil when tended with human care and ingenuity. They bear a blessing that speaks of the divine providence resting over all creation, as the cloud covered the mountain when Moses received the stone tablets of the Law from God (Exod. 24:12–18). And this holiness is the essence of their healing properties: they can help to restore the creature to that goodness which was the initial result of God's creation.

As we grow in spiritual vision, so God is never far from us, even when outer events appear to go very badly for us. The world is seen increasingly to be a sacrament of God's unfailing providence and self-giving love for His creatures. This does not mean that the sacraments of the Church become less important; this understanding in fact deepens their holiness, but at the same time brings the whole world into their orbit. It is our duty and privilege to heal the world – which has in the past suffered immeasurable hurt through the rapacious greed of the human species – and establish harmony and peace among all its creatures. As we bless the world in the name of God, and act that blessing in our daily lives, so the world assumes an increasingly sacramental quality, and in turn heals and purifies all who come into contact with it.

When we have departed from the world of matter at the time of our death, we will see the full sacramental nature of the universe. All that we have handled in love will return to us as a blessing, enabling us to continue the work of healing and restoration in the life beyond death as members, albeit little ones, of the Communion of Saints. God has taught us to see His divine Spirit in such common articles as water, wine, bread and oil. When we have been fully immersed in the sacramental reality of common life, then we will be able to sense the divine presence in all the circumstances of mortal existence. As St Paul says, 'For I am convinced that there is nothing in death or life, in the realm of spirits or superhuman powers, in the world as it is or the world as it shall be, in the forces of the universe, in heights or depths – nothing in all creation that can separate us from the love of God in Christ Jesus our Lord' (Rom. 8:38–9). Every circumstance in life no less than every article we encounter is a way towards healing once we are open to the full thrust of the Holy Spirit. To be sure, some experiences will seem on the surface to be a terrible misfortune and some articles to be frankly noxious. But even in these encounters a larger blessing lies concealed for those who proceed in faith and integrity of purpose. 'Meanwhile, our eyes are fixed not on the things that are seen, but on the things that are unseen: for what is seen passes away; what is unseen is eternal' (2 Cor. 4:18). The sacramental universe links the unseen to the seen, so that the visible may eventually move towards a full participation in eternity. Then there will be no sacraments, but simply one sacrament, a world at rest in God.

8

Prayer and Healing

I wish you all joy in the Lord. I will say it again: all joy be yours. Let your magnanimity be manifest to all. The Lord is near; have no anxiety, but in everything make your requests known to God in prayer and petition with thanksgiving. Then the peace of God, which is beyond our utmost human understanding, will keep guard over your hearts and your thoughts, in Christ Jesus. (Phil. 4:4–7)

Prayer is at the heart of healing; without direct and immediate communion with God, from whom all healing springs, there can be no return to health, no knowledge of wholeness. All healing comes to the creature by the grace of God working through the power of the Holy Spirit. The Spirit's properties are manifold: he is the Lord and giver of life, and also the Spirit of truth, our Advocate who will be with us forever (John 14:26). He is sent in the name of Jesus and he is to teach us everything, recalling to our minds all that Jesus had told the disciples (John 14:26). He is sent to us by the Son from the Father – he issues from the Father as the Spirit of truth – and he bears eternal witness to the nature and the work of the Son (John 15:26). The Spirit of truth not only shows the world where right and wrong and judgement lie (John 16:8), but he also guides those who are open to his fellowship into all the truth; at the present time we, like the disciples, are not able to assimilate all that Jesus could tell us, for the burden is still too great (John 16:12–13). The Spirit of truth does not speak on his own authority, but tells only what he hears, and he informs us of the things that are to be. Above all, he glorifies the Son, for everything that he makes known to us he draws from what is the Son's (John 16:14). In prayer we draw close to the Holy Spirit; in fact although we feel that we are the initiator of our prayers, it is God the Holy Spirit who is the foundation of our praying, the 'ground of our beseeching', as Dame Julian of Norwich puts in (in chapter 41 of *Revelations of Divine Love*). St Paul reminds us that we do not even know how we ought to pray – what it is right to pray for – but through our inarticulate groans, the Spirit himself is pleading for us, and God who searches our inmost being knows what the Spirit means (Rom. 8:26–7). These groans may refer to the gift of ecstatic utterance ('tongues'), but they are even more relevant to the tortured movement into the unknown of the bereft soul groping in the agony of its perplexity.

Prayer is as essential to the well-being of the soul as breathing is to the life of the body. The life-giving power of the Holy Spirit animates the 'inner man' which in turn transforms it into the *vis medicatrix naturae*, the healing force of nature, that restores and renews the physical body. Unfortunately the awareness of unredeemed man is little better than that of a sleep-walker; he is attracted and hypnotized by the surface glitter of daily existence at the expense of the deeper realities of life. In the majority of instances, some immediate crisis of menacing proportions is needed to awaken him to reality, and then he becomes aware of the voice of the Holy Spirit addressing him through his own spirit. The Parable of the Prodigal Son is the immortal paradigm of this awakening to reality: the profligate comes to himself when he sits in penury among the pigs he is tending, because he is at last attentive to the voice of the Spirit within. This voice makes him review his past life with ruthless honesty. Only then can he work towards a recovery of that which has been squandered away in thoughtless debauchery. We listen best to the Spirit of truth when all the usual distractions have departed from us – as they do when we are in dire straits.

They are our good-time friends, like Jesus' disciples who bade a hasty retreat at the time of his betrayal and crucifixion.

Our prayer life starts in the usual run of events with petition and it soon extends to confession. When we pray to God for help in our various difficulties, we are not informing him of anything he does not know. As Jesus says, 'Our Father knows what your needs are before you ask him' (Mat. 6:8). Indeed, he knows the intimate nature of our problems far better than we can understand them, for the Lord does not see as man sees; men judge by appearances, but the Lord judges by the heart (1 Sam. 16:7).

The question arises as to what God's position is in relation to healing. I personally do not doubt that he wills wholeness for all his creatures, but that disease and suffering may sometimes be necessary for wholeness to be attained. The nature of evil's origin, as we have already seen, is a mystery; the great monotheistic religions – Judaism, Christianity and Islam – all agree that God is the sole source of all that is created, whether visible in this world or invisible in the world of psychic relationships. In Isaiah 45:6–7 we read the important doctrine: 'I am the Lord, there is no other; I make the light, I create darkness, author alike of prosperity and trouble. I, the Lord, do all these things.' God himself is, as the greatest mystics have learned, beyond all description, even the categories of good and evil. In his great creative act he has laid the creature open both to beneficial forces that will promote health and happiness, and destructive forces whose end is suffering and annihilation. Which of these is activated depends on the choice, the essential free will of the creature. In our own little world it would seem that the more intricate creatures have evolved from simpler forms of life by genetic mutation and the process of natural selection, whereby those forms most fitted to a particular environment have survived over their less adaptable relatives. The law in the animal world has been disease and mortality long before the development of the human species. The great break-through this human evolution heralded was the emergence of a creature with enormous intellectual potential, able to reflect on himself and his environment, which he could manipulate in full measure, and open to the knowledge of divine reality through his conscious co-operation with the Holy Spirit. In the lower forms of creation that Spirit is an unconscious life-giving power, whereas in man the same Spirit is an agent of sanctification, whereby the inwardly cleansed person may aspire to spiritual knowledge and eventually share in the very being of God, to quote the magnificent text of 2 Peter 1:4 once more.

It is my personal belief that were man fully alive to the creative potentialities of the Holy Spirit, he would not only attain personal health but also bring healing to the rest of the world's creatures. Conversely, when the human psyche breaks down and becomes destructive in tendency, it exerts a disintegrating effect on the other, simpler forms of life. This view has biblical overtones: once man departs from God's grace after the Fall (in Genesis 3), he becomes increasingly alienated from the animal life around him until enmity between the human and the beast is the rule of natural life rather than its exception. On the other hand, the messianic kingdom envisaged in Isaiah 11:6–9 is one of idyllic peace between the various animals with a little child at the head of the procession, leading them all. The little child is a symbol, a sacrament in fact, of a beneficent, completely harmless race of people who give love and service to those around them in marked contrast to the predatory, selfish way of life of unredeemed, unconverted human beings. Therefore, if we pledge ourselves to the preservation of life and the fostering of goodwill among people, we will be open to the healing power of God. If, however, we persist in self-centred, predatory attitudes, we will become vulnerable to the darkness of God, which assumes a terrifyingly winnowing power when it is separated from the divine mercy. Fortunately the process of suffering and destruction can be reversed when we repent and come to ourselves once more (as did the Prodigal Son), confessing our sins to God. The ensuing absolution will set in motion a new life tending to greater wholeness, provided the will is now dedicated to prayer and service instead of the selfish indulgence of the past.

It is the atoning work wrought by the life and death of Christ that assures me categorically of God's will for healing of all his creatures. But his gift of free will precludes any enforcement of his will in the lives of his creatures. Here lies the inevitable limitation set to God's power by his love and courtesy for his rational creatures: he is a father rather than a dictator. Love gives up its very substance for its friend, but it does not overwhelm him with its concern. If commitment is on the one side of the coin of love, freedom blazes emphatically on the other. Love is not clinically detached, neither is it passionately possessive: detachment starves, whereas possessiveness smothers. To find the middle way between these two extremes of human conduct is the great quest of our lives; it is the work of prayer that sheds light on the path of love and illuminates our groping movement towards wholeness.

Petitionary prayer starts with a list of requests made to God with the innocent trust of a child, and as such it is beautiful and in no way to be derided. Sometimes the petition is granted most splendidly, but on other occasions nothing seems to happen, at least as far as we are aware. If we persist in the spiritual life and are not discouraged to the point of quitting by what we consider to be its failure – or more probably our own failure – a deeper consciousness of God gradually dawns upon the questing soul. We begin to understand that the love of God is the beginning and end of all mature prayer, and that the great work is to ease the personal self, or ego, from the centre of our scene, and to set in its place the spiritual self, or soul, with its point of direct contact with God. At this juncture the will of God begins to take precedence in our lives over our own naked will, which is so heavily dominated by our selfish desires that it cannot know what is ultimately best either for us or those we love and serve.

To desire a return to health so as to be a better servant of God would seem on the surface to be entirely praiseworthy, but there may also be undercurrents of self-will and resentment lurking deeper down. In an interesting fashion these attitudes may delay healing no less emphatically than a frank ambivalence to health due to fearfulness or a lack of commitment, such as we considered in the case of the man who had been paralysed for many years before Jesus confronted him directly with his divided mind and made him decide once and for all. It is possible to be all set to do God's

81

work of reclaiming the world from sin, and yet to be so dictatorial about the way the work is to be done that God is slowly excluded from the transaction while one begins to identify oneself subtly with him. We remember in this connection the warning of Jesus,

> Not everyone who calls me 'Lord, Lord' will enter the kingdom of Heaven, but only those who do the will of my Heavenly Father. When that day comes, many will say to me, 'Lord, Lord, did we not prophesy in your name, cast out devils in your name, and in your name perform many miracles?' Then I will tell them to their face, 'I never knew you; out of my sight, you and your wicked ways!'
>
> (Mat. 7:21–3)

The essence of true discipleship to Christ is obedience to the Father and love of the neighbour, who is everyone in our vicinity.

And so prayer, especially in times of adversity, moves from personal petition to full dedication. There is in the end only one petition worthy of man and God, and that repeatedly until the end of time, 'Not as I will, but as thou wilt' (Mat. 26:39). This supreme petition is not simply an affirmation of calm confidence in God's all-embracing providence; it is also the cry of the stricken soul, wounded to the very core of its being beyond human comprehension or creaturely comfort. There is no assurance here, only a desperate self-affirmation in the face of overwhelming psychic darkness. This affirmation of personal integrity is made real by the presence of God, who is never nearer to us than in times of emergency; this intensified awareness of God is a result of our own naked, yet heightened, self-awareness. God is, of course, always present, but we all too often exclude him from the field of our inner vision because we are entranced by the passing show of mortal existence. Imminent disaster concentrates the mind remarkably and has a clearing effect on our usually blurred spiritual vision.

When we are in stillness and rapt dedication before God, contemplating the void from which all being flows, we are open in the fullness of our own being to his presence, whose nature is love. His Spirit then infuses us and sets in motion a healing of a vastly different order to a mere physical relief of suffering. Our minds become re-created in the image of the divine mind, and we start to do the work we were born to accomplish. Similarly, when we are in contemplative communion with God and, at the same time, open in deepest concern to the presence of anyone who is in pain, the Holy Spirit infusing us flows out in love and healing to that person. This is the basis of intercessory prayer, perhaps the apogee of all spiritual healing. Provided the one interceded for is not closed to the grace of God through pride or resentment, he will receive a blessing from God by way of the silent prayer of the person who intercedes for him in the presence of God. It is often the case that the most powerful intercessors are those who are emotionally distant from the people they are helping; emotional involvement can interfere with the Holy Spirit, even deflecting his work of mercy and healing. On the other hand, a warm, though unattached, compassion can effect remarkable healing work through intercession no less than by direct human contact. In this creative attitude of mind the person places himself at God's service instead of being the dominant focus and demanding healing according to what he, in his ignorance, believes is most beneficial for the one in need. We function best spiritually when we are most humble, admitting quite frankly our ignorance and placing ourselves unconditionally at God's service. In the words of the Blessed Virgin at the time of the annunciation, 'Here am I, I am the Lord's servant; as you have spoken, so be it' (Luke 1:38).

Should we therefore not make specific supplications to God? Any dogmatic answer to this question tells us more about the one who gives his opinion than about God's providence. The Holy Spirit will direct us according to the situation; what is of great importance is to get oneself out of the way and be a chaste instrument for God's work. In the celebrated prayer of St Francis of Assisi, the petition that we should be made instruments of his peace, and that we should sow love, pardon, faith, hope, light and joy, is the essence of all our spiritual aspirations. When we can, by the tenor of our lives, manifest some of these qualities – which are in fact fruits of the Holy Spirit – we will receive such healing as is right for us at that time in our lives and give it to others both by direct communication and by distant intercession.

The value of making definite petitions, which is very much the youthful approach to God, is that it centres our own minds on our needs. It has a concentrating effect and leads us to a deeper stillness. In the same way the act of contrition tells God nothing he does not already know, but it serves the valuable psychological and spiritual function of bringing much previously unacknowledged material into a fully aware focus where it can be viewed, in calm confidence, in the conscious presence of God. The additional presence of a trusted friend in this transaction, as in the sacrament of penance, can augment this conscious awareness and help to assure the penitent of God's forgiveness, provided always the will to change is also active. There can be no healing or forgiveness until we are prepared to play our full part in the work. As one grows in the life of prayer, so one's mind becomes more perfectly concentrated on the love of God with the result that all petitions are focused mystically on that timeless moment of union with him. In that space of time, which is in fact outside the temporal sequence, all the requests we have to make, whether personal or intercessory, are transfigured into the supreme petition that we may all be one in God by growing individually and communally into human maturity, measured by nothing less than the full stature of Christ (Eph. 4:13). In this way we concentrate less upon what is disturbed and ill and more on the whole person, whether ourself or someone else.

In healing prayer there are two pitfalls to be avoided: an over-emphasis on bodily cure on the one hand and a virtual dismissal of the body's claims to healing on the other. There is no doubt that a true healing serves to re-create the whole person on a higher level of integration than the clamant ego, which functions on a basis of selfish expediency. While we are rooted in the physical desires, we are imprisoned in a mortal body whose end cannot be other than one of increasing decrepitude that moves inevitably towards death. It is only as the physical desires are transcended that the body can experience its first intimation of resurrection. As St Paul would put it:

Those who live on the level of our lower nature have their outlook formed by it, and that spells death; but those who live on the level of the spirit have the spiritual outlook, and that is life and peace. For the outlook of the lower nature is enmity with God; it is not subject to the law of God; indeed it cannot be: Those who live on such a level cannot possibly please God. (Rom. 8:5–8)

The lower nature, as we have already seen, is not intrinsically evil, for it too is created by God – without it we could not do our daily work. But it is centred on such basic impulses as immediate survival and the satisfaction of its animal desires to the virtual exclusion of all else. The lower nature is an essential servant but a death-dealing master: it, if unchecked, would kill not only others in conflict with it, but eventually itself also. It is for this reason that an emphasis on prayer for bodily restoration is ill-conceived. The right priority is for healing of the entire personality according to God's will.

But it not infrequently happens that a startling bodily healing is the means whereby a previously spiritually dead person comes to life; indeed, the resurrection miracles of Christ are to be seen as much in this light as in terms of a mere prolongation of life and postponement of death. If we were to exclude the physical healings from the Gospel accounts, we would have little to show of Jesus' burning compassion as well as his charismatic presence. It is said in Mark 1:14–15 that after John the Baptist had been arrested Jesus came into Galilee proclaiming the Gospel of God: 'The time has come; the kingdom of God is upon you; repent, and believe the Gospel.' In this respect Jesus is both the messenger and the message. The healings of Jesus were signs of the imminence of the Kingdom. The body, while not to be equated with the whole personality, is neither to be denigrated, let alone dismissed. The Word did not disdain the flesh of incarnation any more than the womb of the Blessed Virgin. Since human awareness is often limited to the flesh, it is right that in most instances healing should commence on a purely physical level. Nor need this healing be dramatically charismatic; a cure based on orthodox medical practice can be equally radical in its deeper repercussions to one who is attaining a degree of spiritual awareness. The dedication and skill of the doctors and the compassion and care of the nursing staff may make deep inroads into the previously obtuse awareness of a patient who comes to himself while in hospital.

Some of the most outstanding testimonies to the power of prayer are seen in patients who are undergoing major surgical procedures. The patient seems often to be endued with an inner strength and outer resilience that amazes those who are tending him. Recovery is often remarkably rapid considering the gravity of the condition, and the amount of pain and distress is much less than would have been expected. The basis of this prayer, it should be reiterated, is not that there should be a rapid recovery but simply that the Spirit of God should infuse the one in need and fill him with renewed life and purpose. The end is God's will, not ours; we are the means whereby the will of God can be actualized. 'In stillness and in staying quiet, there lies your strength' (Isa. 30:15); in this instance the Israelites chose obsessive political manipulation rather than calm trust in God – the essence of the faith that heals – and they were mercilessly routed by their foes. Activism is the bane of humanistic endeavour; to do something is almost a means of self-justification, and the result is more often dissatisfaction than constructive work. Activity, by contrast, is the way of the Spirit-infused person: his first action is prayer, our most noble work, which is followed by the inflow of purpose and the calm, carefully considered assessment of the task in hand. In other words, faith is followed by good works in which the divine purpose guides and strengthens the human initiative. This divine–human collaboration is the essence of all constructive activity and is the culmination as well as the fulfilment of the healing process. In Jesus Christ the two natures, the divine and the human, are perfectly united and aligned, so that he can proclaim, and at the same time make manifest, the imminence of the kingdom of God; here healing is both complete and universal. 'For as the heavens are higher than the earth, so are my ways higher than your ways, and my thoughts than your thoughts' (Isa. 55:9).

In the deeper approach to healing prayer an especially plausible reaction is the temptation to feel ashamed that one is so limited by the body in its affliction as to be virtually impotent, whereas if one were truly spiritual one could lift oneself above the distress of the moment to eternal communion with the divine. This is a dangerous attitude that smacks of gnosticism, a heresy that exalts the spirit which is good, while denigrating the body which, being material, is considered evil. There may well be mental, meditative techniques that can lift a person above bodily awareness, but except as a temporary expedient to transcend severe pain while a special service has to be undertaken, these are not to be recommended as a way towards healing. Christ himself did not flinch from a full participation in the psychic darkness that envelops this world any more than he evaded the physical agony of the cross. By immersing himself freely in the pain and darkness of the world he lifted it up and commenced its healing as well as the healing of the countless millions of creatures bowed down under that darkness. We too have to wrestle with the angel of apparent darkness, as Jacob did in his mysterious encounter with the divine presence in the depths of the night, before we can claim our blessing: a transformed consciousness and an ability to serve God and man in a completely new awareness. This awareness is no longer limited by the ego with its desires of personal recompense, but is now transpersonal with the desire for universal healing. One does not lift oneself above one's affliction so much as go patiently and with courage through it, so that the thing of darkness which was previously of forbidding intensity is now accepted as part of oneself. Only then can a healing be initiated that lasts.

This acceptance of adversity, which is very much a part of the healing process, is not to be confused with a passive, spineless resignation to what is believed to be the will of God. Acceptance looks positively for healing, seeing in the words of St Paul in Romans 8:28, that all things work together for good for those who love God. Each moment of life, terrifying as it may appear on the surface, has an underlying value to be gauged in the future when our vision is no longer clouded by the confusion of the present, but can encompass the larger scheme of spiritual growth. In this exalted frame of mind we can work together with God in the transmutation of evil to good rather than merely depend on God to release us from the evil around us. Such a release would be at most only a temporary expedient, and in due course the darkness would return, persisting until it was encountered in faith and courage in the name of the Lord. He is with us always, to the end of time (Mat. 28:20), and in his presence there is the consummation of all things to the divine essence. It is in this spirit that prayer works most perfectly and restores all that is disfigured and malaligned to the divine image in which it was originally created.

The man of prayer is a sacrament of the newly risen race of people who will know God in the depths of their being. In the words of Jeremiah 31:33: 'This is the covenant which I shall make with Israel after those days, says the Lord; I will set my law within them and write it on their hearts; I will become their God and they shall become my people.' They will no longer need to teach one another to know God, for all of them, high and low alike, will know him in their cleansed souls, now in direct communion with the Most High. Thus prayer that starts as a simple conversation with God in child-like trust, broadens and deepens to a complete self-giving to God in which an inward renewal is attained. This puts all our mundane conceptions of healing into the class of childish demands as compared with the total healing that God has in store for us. But every step on the way has its own validity and is not to be derided, any more than the view of life we had when we were young is to be dismissed as worthless as we attain the greater wisdom of life's experience. The rungs of the ladder on which we have ascended to the heights are all precious in themselves and should be blessed in retrospect as we move ever upwards on the path of charity that leads to God himself. His Son is indeed the way that we follow to the glorious end, which is the beatific vision.

9

The Gift of Healing

He went around the whole of Galilee, teaching in the synagogues, preaching the gospel of the Kingdom, and curing whatever illness or infirmity there was among the people. His fame reached the whole of Syria; and sufferers from every kind of illness, racked with pain, possessed by devils, epileptic, or paralysed, were all brought to him, and he cured them. Great crowds also followed him, from Galilee and the Ten Towns, from Jerusalem and Judaea, and from Transjordan. (Mat. 4:23–5)

The gift of healing comes from God; indeed the agent of healing is the Holy Spirit. The human instrument brings that Spirit fully down to earth and initiates a process of restoration that accompanies him wherever he goes. It therefore follows that the two requirements in the healing ministry are an openness to God and a deep concern for one's fellow creatures. These prerequisites are summed up in the two great commandments: loving God with all our being, and loving our neighbour as ourself. This latter clause requires, and indeed assumes, self-love also; an acceptance of oneself and one's various difficulties and inadequacies with a warm-hearted sense of humour, and a gratitude to the Creator that one has been given life with its infinite possibilities despite these inadequacies of character. As soon as we can accept ourselves in this open-hearted spirit, we can forget ourselves in service to God and our fellows, and at last the Holy Spirit can start his life-enhancing work in us and then through us to those around us. The gift of healing is in essence an ability to make rapid and deep soul-relationships – psychic empathy it could be called – with other people, and then becoming the channel through which the Holy Spirit can perform his renewing and sanctifying work. The mere psychic empathy will effect the transfer of spiritual power from one person to another, and some of those with a healing gift are neither believers in God nor especially admirable people. If they remain at a spiritually debased level they can progressively drain those around them, and in the end cause harm. This is why a gift of healing must be a part of a deeper spirituality, one in which the person offers it, and indeed himself, unconditionally to God and to his fellow men. His reward is not pecuniary but purely the joy of seeing one who 'was dead and has come back to life, was lost and is found' (Luke 15:32).

Such a person is a focus for the healing power of the Holy Spirit wherever he finds himself. He does not need to display any characteristic gestures to implement the flow of the Holy Spirit, since he is always an instrument of God's peace and a constant source of pardon, hope and joy. The basis of such a healing faculty is the assiduous practice of prayer. This prayer, it should be noted, is not one for healing powers to be made manifest in one's life, but simply an unfailing awareness of the divine presence within one's being and around one in whatever situation one finds oneself. In other words, contemplative communion with the Most High is the foundation of an authentic healing ministry. One need not ask God for the gift so much as be worthy to receive it, for when it is given it has to be dispensed without condition, so that one's very life is no longer a purely private matter but is the life that Christ lives in one. There is no glamour in a truly healing ministry; there is only unmitigated service that is lightened by the power of discernment given one as the work proceeds. But such a life of dedication to God and the brethren is the height of spirituality, compared with which all worldly rewards are meretricious dross. It was for this service that we were conceived, and each in his own way has to fulfil it in his life no matter what his particular trade or occupation may be. A person serving behind a shop counter can be a minister of healing when he flows out in concern to the customer and gives his whole attention to serving him and satisfying his demands in gracious solicitude. When we yield of ourselves spontaneously to a stranger in difficulties and help him on his way, we are performing a healing act far in excess of the superficial assistance we may be affording. We are giving him not only expert advice but also something of the spirit within us. This is a high interpretation of the Parable of the Good Samaritan, who healed the stranger fallen among thieves and battered by them no less significantly than the inn-keeper to whom he later entrusted the wounded man.

It cannot be stated too often that the essence of healing is an attitude of quiet, unobtrusive hope that emanates from the humble soul shriven of the dross of material desire by the winnowing experiences of life. It is the second simplicity that we all have to know if we are to enter the kingdom of heaven as a little child. The wisdom of the serpent and the harmlessness of the dove that Jesus enjoins on his disciples are the qualities displayed by such a heavenly person: the wisdom comes from God and is transmitted to the humble soul who has no regard for proprietary rights, but is an untroubled agent of all God's gifts to those around him. There is, in this respect, an important difference between a virtuous person and one who is holy. The virtuous person, excellent in his own way, keeps well within the demands of the moral law and is a fine, reliable citizen and colleague provided those around him are equally trustworthy. But there will usually be a tendency to judge others uncharitably if they fail to attain his high standards. This was the essence of the spiritual failure of the Pharisee who thanked God that he was so much better than other people, especially the wretched tax-gatherer who stood next to him (Luke 18:9–14). Virtue can all too easily become a god in its own right and exclude the Living God of love; the same can apply to even the finest religion, as the world's history shows all too often.

A holy person, by contrast, brings God closer to all the people he meets. He does this by the spiritual radiance that emanates from him. By nature a holy man is simple in his life-style – even if he possesses considerable wealth – and

humble in his attitude to all whom he encounters in his daily
rounds. This humility is a transparency of the personality so
that other people, no matter how ignorant they may appear
to the world, are accepted unconditionally for what they are,
children of God. The result is that the humble person can
learn something from everyone he meets and from every
circumstance in life, no matter how unpropitious it may
appear. The secret of relating deeply to other people is an
attitude of self-giving to the moment at hand with as few
preconceptions and prejudices as possible to cloud the vision
and colour the judgement. When one enters the ministry of
healing in such an attitude of self-abandonment to the divine
providence – to quote the title of de Caussade's spiritual
classic to which allusion has already been made – the Holy
Spirit flows through one and initiates the essential healing
work. The more one tries to assist the work of the Holy Spirit,
the more one interposes one's own will in that work, and at
once an obstruction is set up. Just as the finest personal
relationships depend on an activation of the souls within the
people involved, so the gift of healing works most effectively
when the souls of all involved vibrate in harmony together.
A holy person, being close to God, brings the Holy Spirit
down to the consciousness of all whom he encounters.

Holiness is something more than mere virtue: it is an attitude of complete harmlessness and love. It is a divine simplicity in which a knife-sharp discrimination is developed. This
simplicity is no mere naivety – a capacity to be deceived
because one's knowledge of the world is defective. It is, on
the contrary, an intuitive grasp of the whole of life, informed
by the undistorted action of the Holy Spirit working in the
full personality, but executed in unselfconscious charity. In
fact there is only one fundamental act of will that is needed
for the healing ministry: to place oneself unconditionally at
God's service and to practise his presence in absolute stillness.
In this state one is an immaculate vehicle for the Spirit of
God, and a healing will be given that touches and renews the
soul. This in turn may affect the body also, but here other
considerations must be given due weight: the extent of bodily
disease, the person's will to be healed, his attitude to life, and
the fact of human mortality. We can never demand physical

results from a healing session; all we can look for is spiritual renewal. Following in its wake – and sometimes dramatically preceding it – there may be a physical healing also.

All this indicates that a healing gift comes from God but that it is our great privilege to use it to his honour and glory and to the benefit of those around us, our perpetual neighbours in this life and that which is to follow. The difference between a person who has a natural gift of healing, but whose aspirations are essentially selfish and predatory, and a true minister of spiritual healing does not lie in the source or nature of the healing power. All power comes from God, 'who makes his sun rise on good and bad alike, and sends the rain on the honest and the dishonest' (Mat. 5:45). There is only one Holy Spirit who gives life and potency to all the creation. Whether that life becomes a blessing or a curse, and whether the potency is creative or destructive depends on the use put to it by the creature. Spiritual gifts can assume a demonic character if the honour is appropriated by those who possess them; we remember once more the statement of Christ that not everyone who calls him Lord will enter the kingdom of heaven even if he displays miraculous powers in his name. It is those who do the Father's will who alone will enter (Mat. 7:21–3). This will is mirrored in Christ's life on earth, and therefore the closer our own lives approach his life, the more perfect will be our healing presence.

To spell this out in greater detail, Jesus never took credit for his powers, but gave acknowledgement always to the Father. He gained nothing personally from his work – except, of course, an increasing reputation for holiness and spiritual understanding. He coveted neither money nor political power, neither social advantage nor academic honours. His work was to herald the kingdom of God in the world, for which purpose he was prepared to sacrifice his own life on the cross of human despair, so that even despair could be resurrected in a fresh hope of eternal love. Indeed, there is only one quality worthy of desire: love, which is the very nature of God. Love alone prevails when all else has undergone the attrition of ageing and mortal death. Therefore the gift of healing is used to its best advantage in a person filled with self-giving love, whose only desire is to save what is lost, as Jesus said in connection with the repentant tax-gatherer, Zacchaeus (Luke 19:10). There are no techniques of spiritual healing, only the assiduous practice of contemplative prayer and a life dedicated to the service of one's fellows.

It must be emphasized, however, that this selfless devotion to God and our fellow creatures includes ourselves also; the love of one's neighbour is to equal that of oneself. Until one is healthy in body as well as in mind, heart and soul, one will not be able to do one's work effectively in the world. Therefore a balanced diet and attractive living conditions, far from being an indulgence to the flesh, are prerequisites for an effective healing ministry. Likewise, there is a limit to the work any one person can do; if that limit is exceeded a physical and mental breakdown will inevitably follow. Therefore one must learn not only how and when to say 'No', but also how to delegate one's work to other servers on the way. To admit one's limitations is a practical exercise in humility, and to drop one's cloak over the shoulders of those who are to continue the work when one is no longer available oneself, in the manner of Elijah and Elisha (1 Kings 19:19–21), is the acid test of spiritual generosity.

It follows therefore that no healing ministry worthy of its name can ignore the teaching aspect. The person seeking healing should be instructed about the levels of the human personality: body, mind and soul with special emphasis on the glory of the spirit in man which is in communion with the Holy Spirit of God. He should also be taught that true faith is an unobstructed openness to God, however he may be conceived, and not an absolute reliance on any person, no matter how gifted he may be. The informed healing minister is a sacrament: Christ works through his hands and speaks from the teaching of his lips. The essence of both giving and receiving healing is a suspension of judgement, so that one becomes once more a little child to whom alone is the kingdom of God available. This judgement includes both credulity and incredulity: the Holy Spirit's work is hindered as much by attempts to spur it on as by a closed attitude of mind to all categories of thought that transcend the narrow bounds of reason. This incidentally implies no contempt for rational thought, but simply an acknowledgement that there is more in heaven and earth than are contained in the tenets of science and philosophy, at least as far as these have developed up to the present time. As we learn more about spiritual healing and the laws that govern it, so the bounds of human reason will be extended, and the scientific world-view, which is basically sound enough, will be broadened by the inclusion of new data.

The secret of constructive living is balance – a balance between body and soul, between mind and heart, so that each is given its due rewards and taught its austere responsibilities. It is in this frame of reference that the various agencies of healing work in greatest harmony – medical science, psychotherapy, the charismatic healing gift and the sacraments of the Church. The uniting principles are an attitude of humility in all who minister and an assiduous practice of prayer. This acts, amongst other ways, to get the selfish ego out of its place of dominance so that it can effect its proper work of service to God and our fellow creatures. We generally do our best work, whether in the realm of relationships or in artistic or scientific creativity, when we are least aware of ourselves; it is a matter once more of the life we live no longer being merely our own life, but the life that Christ lives in us. His openness to the Father is ours also, and remarkable feats become attainable to us according to our capacity to contain and work with the Holy Spirit. It is in this context that a healthy body, an accomplished mind and an ardent heart find their greatest value. An intellectually articulate person can communicate more effectively than one who is illiterate, just as a person of warm, affectionate nature is more easily approachable than one who is cold and withdrawn. But neither intellectual mastery nor overflowing affection will effect a healing ministry; for this the Holy Spirit is mandatory, and as Jesus tells Nicodemus, that spirit blows, like the wind, where he wills; we can hear the sound but we do not know where he comes from nor where he is going (John 3:8). The most unlikely people may be chosen for this work, while the traditional religionist may be completely unresponsive to the flow of God's Spirit.

Some healers of a spiritualistic turn of mind believe that their gift comes from discarnate sources in the life beyond death, and often claim to know the identity of their inspirer (or 'control', or 'guide', as it is usually called). Such claims need not be dismissed out of hand; we know too little about these mysterious matters to enjoy the luxury of dogmatic utterances for or against them. The doctrine of the Communion of Saints can be invoked to include such discarnate entities as once walked our earth as we do at present. But in fact this is of secondary importance; what matters is God and his work among us. What means he chooses to bring his Spirit down to us is not primarily our business. We tend, as humans, to become so enmeshed in the glamour of personality, whether of this world or the next, that we all too easily lose contact with the Source of all being. Furthermore, a reliance on a discarnate personality can have a stultifying effect on our own powers of discrimination. Therefore, although it seems highly probable that intermediaries exist in the psychic and spiritual worlds that interpenetrate our own, and some of these may well be true messengers of God's Spirit for our education and healing, it is right that our spiritual sight should be lifted up to God himself in prayer rather than diverted to discourse with psychic entities, no matter how uplifting their teaching may be. If their teaching is authentically spiritual it will bring us closer to God, so that we will not have to devote our time to communicating with them. The most serious criticism of psychic communication in general is its trivial nature, added to which, of course, there is the danger of infiltration of malign psychic influences emanating from mischievous entities. The greatest psychic powers cannot be compared in excellence to the sacraments of a living religious tradition and the ageless wisdom that has proceeded from the lips and lives of its saints. The effect of charismatic power will soon be dissipated if it is not accompanied by a spiritual teaching of high potency that changes the very life of the person desiring to be healed.

The same principles are true of healing services in a church as part of its regular liturgy. The mere laying-on of hands at the altar rail is not enough; it must be accompanied by an authoritative teaching ministry aided, if possible, by a counselling service. In this way the mind is brought into the full ambience of God's healing. The Holy Spirit works in these manifold ways, and if the assistance of those who are medically qualified is also available, a very powerful healing ministry is afforded to those in need. Nowadays the concept of holistic medicine is current; it includes, in addition to the healing arms already mentioned, a stress on diet and meditation and sometimes also such unorthodox therapies as homeopathy, herbalism and acupuncture, whose scientific basis remains obscure. It is probable that a strongly psychic basis attends these forms of treatment, and in addition there is a very close emotional empathy between the practitioner and his patient. We should be open to all advances in the healing ministry, no matter where they originate. But our discernment must always be active and alert. The psychic mode of communication is much more intimate than the intellectual approach used by the medical scientist. It depends on a close rapport between therapist and patient. Therefore the moral integrity of the therapist is especially important, since he can easily impose his prejudices on the mind of his patient. Repeating the advice of Jesus, we need the wisdom of the serpent and the harmlessness of the dove in all our healing work, and nowhere is this more true than in those therapies with a psychic basis.

In a healing ministry the dangers especially to be recognized are a tendency to dominate the lives of those who come for help and a zeal to prove the ways of God by virtue of the healings accomplished. These 'ways of God' accord with our own understanding rather than with God's will. Therefore such a limited view will tend to attribute a failure of physical healing either to a lack of faith or deep, unacknowledged guilt for past sins. But God sees differently from man: we see the surface while God looks into the heart. When a person's failure to get well is summarily attributed to his lack of faith, insult is often added to the injury he has already sustained. In such a heartless accusation it is faith in the healer that is questioned rather than trust in God; the healer sees the failure to respond as a tacit impugnment of his own gift and is thereby diminished as a person. It follows therefore that we should not enter a healing ministry until we ourselves are at least fairly well integrated as people and do not need success or the plaudits of others to sustain our rather shaky identity. Likewise, there should be no financial charge for a spiritual gift. If a thankful person wishes to make a contribution he need not necessarily be deterred, since it can also be a healing act to receive from someone overflowing with gratitude. It is true that happiness lies more in giving than in receiving (Acts 20:35), but there is a peculiar graciousness and humility in being open to the praise and gifts of others. The important requirement is, of course, to give the glory to God, so that the praise falls away from oneself as easily as water off a duck's back, and we can thank God in unison with the healed one for all that has been achieved. The reward of having a healing gift is to see the afflicted person rise from despair to joy; compared with this, money is irrelevant.

Since it is preferable not to depend for one's subsistence on spiritual gifts, it follows that one's living should be earned in some other way, if this is at all practicable. This approach has the added advantage of taking the one who ministers healing out of the rather restricting confines of his work into the greater world where he can consort for at least a part of his time with vigorous, healthy people. The constant demands of the sick and the emotionally distraught cannot but have a depressing effect on those who minister to them on a spiritual level. It is for this reason that a complete break in the atmosphere of surrounding gloom is necessary each day in the lives of those involved in the work of healing and counselling. The toll of psychic depletion (evidenced in Jesus' ministry when he felt the power leave him after the woman with haemorrhages had touched him quite deliberately, as recounted in Mark 5:25–34) can be enormous if the power is not constantly replenished by a break in the routine of work, especially when this is attended by prayer.

When we study the ministry of Jesus, especially as described in Luke's gospel, we cannot fail to note his ability of escaping from the pressure of the heavy demands made on him, not only by the infirm but also, at times, by his rather obtuse, insensitive disciples. When he was alone, he was in deep prayer (Luke 3:21, 5:16, 6:12). He could also pray alone in the company of his disciples (Luke 9:18, 9:28–9, 11:1, 22:41), whom, no doubt, he taught the way to a deeper, more comprehensive prayer life than the mere repetition of traditional sentences that so often passes for prayer and is in fact the betrayal and finally the death of a living faith. Real prayer is an elevation of the mind to God so that we can commune with him in rapt attention and in deepest love. Sometimes Jesus took his disciples with him where they could be alone in the noiseless tranquillity of nature before the crowds caught up with them and their outer peace was disrupted (Mark 3:7, 6:45). The inner peace of Christ, however, was never shattered, for he was in constant communion with his Father. It is thus that all who are involved in a ministry of healing should proceed in their private lives. When they too can know an inner peace that does not need results or acclaim to substantiate it, they have attained the apogee of their healing work. No more do they have to justify God's ways to man; they simply bring into manifestation the love of God who uses the whole world as a healing sacrament for our benefit.

The secret of spirituality, from which all healing gifts derive, is a simplicity of life-style (including the food we eat), openness to the advent of each new day and all it brings with it, and empathy with all who communicate with us. There is a joy inherent in all life when we can give of ourselves fully to it, and in that joy a radiance emanates from us to all our neighbours. This is the heart of our healing ministry: it is a gift of love to all who will receive.

10

The Problem of the Unhealed

And so, to keep me from being unduly elated by the magni-ficence of such revelations, I was given a sharp physical pain which came as Satan's messenger to bruise me; this was to save me from being unduly elated. Three times I begged the Lord to rid me of it, but his answer was: 'My grace is all you need; power comes to its full strength in weakness'. (2 Cor. 12:7–9)

No account of the ministry of healing is authentic unless it deals with the painful and very pertinent question of those who apparently fail to be healed. These, at least on the surface, would seem to include a considerable proportion of those who seek spiritual help when the scientific methods have failed to cure them. It is noteworthy, in this respect, that the orthodox doctor tends to remember his failures, whereas the unorthodox practitioners of healing usually regale the world with impressive accounts of their successes. The not inconsiderable number of people who fail to benefit from their diverse ministries are summarily swept from public view under a carpet of oblivion. Indeed, we still look for the controlled type of trial in heterodox healing methods that is now the rule in assessing drug and other orthodox therapies. Anecdotes of success are not an acceptable alternative to the sound, probing analysis of results that is taken for granted in scientific circles. And yet is this the heart of healing?

When we sift out those people who have never truly played their part in co-operating with God, through a lack of humility, faith or commitment, there is still a considerable number of earnest sufferers who have failed to respond in any manifest way to the full ministry of healing. These are a source of constant embarrassment to the agencies of healing that pride themselves on a near perfect restoration to health of all who consult them: worse still, this failure calls into question either God's power or his love. If prayer remains so blatantly unheard that no response appears to have been made, the questing human being will have considerable difficulty in locating God's concern in the world.

The answer to this problem appears to reside in the universal prevalence of hatred and sin. We are indeed parts of one body, as St Paul puts it (Eph. 4:25), and the very concept of individual healing is selfish and indeed unreal except in the context of a resurrection of the world from the domination of the powers of darkness to the effulgent radiance of the uncreated light of God. It is in this frame of reference that the conversion of all people from the way of selfish abandon to the challenge of growth into the fullness of humanity, as shown in Christ, is constantly before us and is our most urgent priority for the healing of the world. While even one person is in hell, not even the greatest saint can be truly in heaven. Thus it is well said by Pascal that Christ will be in agony until the end of the world, and we dare not, like the three disciples with him in Gethsemane, fall asleep. It is, in a very intimate way, a privilege for those who love Christ most to share this vigil. In this frame of mind St Paul writes (in Col. 1:24): 'It is my happiness to suffer for you. This is my way of helping to complete, in my poor human flesh, the full tale of Christ's afflictions still to be endured, for the sake of his body which is the church.' The suffering is something more than a gesture of solidarity, important as this may be in a heedless world where it is never easy to stand up for righteousness' sake and be counted amongst those who are prepared to give up their very lives for what they believe most passionately. The suffering that St Paul underwent as described so starkly in 2 Cor. 11:23–7, is merely a prelude to the deeper pain he mentions in relation to his undying concern for the sufferings of the infant Christian congregations he had helped to establish, and which is mentioned in the last verses of that chapter: he shares the weakness of the frail, the indignation of those who are made to stumble, and the fear of those who are persecuted. In this last consideration we remember the fugitives from totalitarian tyranny in our own time. Those who shielded them even to their own death are inscribed among the saints of humanity. By their wounds we are healed in eternity, as prophesied in Isaiah 53 – the wounds of those who learnt to forgive their persecutors even as they were hounded to death are in this respect added to those of their protectors who died in fidelity to the truth.

All this means in effect that pain has its own deeper understanding to contribute, and we will not be released from its bondage until we have assimilated its full message; we are to grow into nothing less than the full stature of Christ, not merely on a private, individualistic level but, more pertinently, in communion with all humanity. And the end of that growth is a raising of all life to the full knowledge of God. Until the last trace of egoistic isolation has been removed from us, we will neither be healed nor bring healing to others. The saints of the world have accepted suffering vicariously in order to share the otherwise intolerable burdens that continue to afflict individual men and women. This sharing of pain is not a willed, exhibitionistic gesture, but an intuitive response to the demands of love. As Jesus taught us, there is no greater love than this, that a man should lay down his life for his friends (John 15:13), and the saint, in spontaneous imitation of Christ (whether or not he calls himself a Christian), accepts all mankind – indeed the whole of creation – as his friend.

None of us is to survive in his present form; death is indeed the gateway to a fuller life that brings us closer to the knowledge of eternity. What is important in this transitory life on earth is our growth into fuller relationship with one another. Jesus, in the somewhat enigmatic Parable of the Unjust Steward, teaches that even the unjust who work astutely to repair, however inadequately, some of the wrong they have done, may be received by friends into an eternal home in the life beyond death where money is a thing of the past (Luke 16:9). We will never know, in our present state of spiritual consciousness, the service rendered by the saintly unhealed in lifting the burden of pain from their uninstructed brethren who are spiritually blind.

As we have already noted, this service is not rendered as an ego-centred gesture of spiritual largesse; on the contrary, it is given to God in humble trust, so that even a little suffering can be alleviated by the action of psychic empathy which precedes the release of the pain of the world into God's providence. In the deepest psychic communion the pain can be exchanged, and the saint can act as a substitute, as Christ did for our sins. The suffering is given in trust and prayer to God, in whom it is transfigured in glory. The atoning reconciliation effected cosmically by Christ is confirmed and realized on a more personal level by the saints who come close to their afflicted brethren to shelter them under their mantle of care. As they present our suffering to God in humble trust, so the first steps are taken towards the transmutation of that suffering into purpose and eventually into radiant joy – the joy of the knowledge of God's eternal presence in our lives.

I am sure there is no divine satisfaction in surveying the baneful effects of sin and gluttony; on the contrary, it is God's will that we should be healed, but for this to be accomplished, we too must play our part. The saints of this world, without premeditation and in sprightly spontaneity, fulfil what St Paul calls the law of Christ, that we should help one another in carrying these heavy loads, in bearing one another's burdens (Gal. 6:2). Once the saints of humanity have helped discharge an intolerable incubus of darkness, we baser mortals are strengthened to play our part also, in so doing rising visibly closer to our own sanctification. Martyrdom is not chosen as a path towards self-exaltation; it is assumed in the slow, often halting, always unobtrusive progress of a life, often stumbling over mortal weaknesses, which is nevertheless moving unceasingly to complete service to God. And the will of God is that we should all, in our own way, come to share in his very being (2 Pet. 1:4).

'A precious thing in the Lord's sight is the death of those who die faithful to him' (Ps. 116:15); that faith is tested and purified in the fiery crucible of suffering, and to those who have passed the test is given that unsurpassable privilege of helping their brethren, whether in this life or the next. In this statement there is a double truth, a reversible privilege. Those who have passed the test have moved towards sanctification whether they are still with us in the flesh or have passed on into the life beyond mortal death. If they are still with us in this world, their witness illuminates our lives with fresh purpose, while their intercessions help the earth-bound dead to quit their hellish isolation and progress to an intermediary purgatorial state. On the other hand, if the saints of our time have died, they take their place among their fellows in the life beyond death: here they assist us on our way while helping to release their earth-bound brethren in the life they now share. Both these actions are performed by intercessory prayer. In this respect the great Communion of Saints includes us in our feeble works no less than the great ones in the after-life. All who are not against God are for him, and the test of sincerity is how much our own lives reflect the love of Christ in our attitude to the world and especially to those around us, whom Jesus would have identified as our neighbours. No ministry of healing that remains oblivious of this higher calling of mankind is worthy of its name.

This being so, the question arises whether there should be any ministry of relief and physical cure at all if suffering plays such an important part in the development of a saint's character and his ministry in the world. The answer would appear to be that God works increasingly towards the healing of his creation; what he made has fallen from its highest potentiality through its own imperfect will, a lapse augmented no doubt by the malign influence of psychic powers in the world beyond death. Of those we have already spoken in connection with deliverance from evil. But we believe that man is to rise to an even greater height of excellence when his chastened will acts in responsible co-operation with the divine will. In Dame Julian's immortal words, 'Sin is behovable, but all shall be well, and all shall be well, and all manner of thing shall be well' (*Revelations of Divine Love*, chapter 27). It would seem that the forgiveness of sin, when sought with true repentance and earnest intent to begin a new way of life, brings an experience of love into the heart of the sinner that changes the course of his future career. It is in this way that holiness transfigures basic virtue, so that a good man may now attain the stature of a saint.

If all this is placed in the context of the ministry of healing as the world understands it, the little cures and improvements that we bear witness to in our private lives serve to whet our appetites for a greater healing. This is to have a world-wide scope, so that the grace of God which we personally have known may now be available to all who suffer. In this greater healing some will play their part as renewed, active, healthy agents, a glorious testimony to the powers of healing in the world, ranging from the medical to the charismatic. But others, like St Paul whose experience of failure in healing prefixed this chapter, have to bear the pain of suffering and even martyrdom, so that others may begin to glimpse the first light of spiritual day. But in the end all shall be well. Christ gave of his riches so that the world's poverty might be remedied, to the end that all might share in the munificence of God. The little saints follow his example and help to shed his light according to the will of God.

There are other deeper considerations also: some people attribute a failure of healing – especially when the sufferer is born irremediably defective – to a great sin committed in a past existence, perhaps here on earth or else in some other dimension of experience. Here we can in all humility admit only ignorance. Suffice to say that there is no scientific proof of pre-existence, any more than of a life of the personality when the body perishes, and we have to come to our own conclusions about these greater mysteries of existence. But an obvious danger of attributing present distress to actions in the distant past beyond personal recall is that a judgemental attitude is likely to ensue as well as a somewhat detached, even fatalistic, approach to the suffering of others. It is all too easy to dismiss such pain as a lesson to be learnt or a necessary punishment to be endured, and then to move past on the other side of the road of life, like the priest and the Levite who ignored the plight of the man robbed and beaten on the way from Jerusalem to Jericho (Luke 10:29–37). It may well be that a permanent impediment is here to teach us a vital lesson in humility, patience and forebearance, but what is important is that the thorn in the flesh (to quote once more St Paul's experience in failure to be healed) is seen to be a means of spiritual growth and not simply a deadening incubus placed on the person as an inexorable punishment for some sin of which he is ignorant and therefore cannot truly repent. We have to learn, as St Paul did, how our power comes to full strength in weakness.

No one could accuse St Paul of a vacillating faith or a feeble resolve. Indeed his activity was probably strengthened by the handicap he was obliged to bear. We act most wisely when we do not allow ourselves to be side-tracked into absorbing speculations about the ultimate cause of an illness or an impediment. Such theoretical considerations can indeed be diverting as well as ego-enhancing, but they take us away from what is of far greater import: an understanding of what the present situation, unpleasant as it may be, is telling us about our own disposition and that of the others who are involved in the trouble. This is the way of progressive self-knowledge, and if we persist fearlessly in complete, unshuttered awareness of the moment in hand, much of the past will be revealed to us as well. This deeper revelation will come to us as we are ready to receive it. Thus, although there is probably more to a person's history than we can glimpse in our present state of spiritual immaturity, we are advised to keep our eyes in one-pointed concentration on the present moment, which also is the point of intersection of time with eternity.

There are certain physical laws which, no doubt, are reflections of the spiritual law of life. If a person loses an eye or a limb, he cannot grow a new one. Certainly modern medical practice can ameliorate the loss with variable degrees of success: some prostheses can replace amputated limbs with remarkable functional performance, but they have no feeling in them. At present nothing can replace the sight of an eye or the hearing of an ear: once these sense organs are irreparably damaged there is only blindness or deafness to anticipate. Likewise the death of a beloved friend is irreversible. Those who seek for comfort in spiritualistic communication are retarding their own spiritual growth and probably interfering with that of the loved one also. Life moves on, both here and in the realms beyond death; our memories are precious, but they must be the inspiration to new work in the time left to us here and now. If we wallow in them to the exclusion of practical endeavour for the future, they become our prison and ultimately our tomb. We have to learn to accept God's 'No' to our present schemes of success in order to come to his greater 'Yes' for our growth into union with him. That was the message given to St Paul after his prayers for bodily healing were left unanswered. 'Hence I am well content, for Christ's sake, with weakness, contempt, persecution, hardship and frustration; for when I am weak, then I am strong (2 Cor. 12:10).

While we have the rude health and exuberant activity of youth, we should enjoy our life in all its fullness. Not to have tasted of the manifold fruits of existence that God has prepared for us is a sin rather than an act of commendable renunciation, for it implies a denial of the life we have been given. In the boundless grace of a vigorous, healthy body we are to affirm every moment of our existence, remembering the high privilege it is to be born human: we embrace an animal body with a spiritual mind, so bringing together the profligate fecundity of nature with the boundless providence of the divine. We are God's priests, and our supreme function is to consecrate ourselves and all the world to his service and glory. Each moment of aware human life is a sacrament in its own right, provided we lift it up to God.

'Remember your Creator in the days of your youth, before the time of trouble comes and the years draw near when you will say, "I see no purpose in them." Remember him before the sun and the light of the day give place to darkness' (Eccles. 12:1–2), or as Jesus was later to add, 'While daylight lasts we must carry on the work of him who sent me; night comes, when no one can work. While I am in the world, I am the light of the world' (John 9:4–5). The wonder of it all is this: if we remember God with thanksgiving in the days of our active life when happiness surrounds us, he will be with us even more emphatically when the inevitable shadows of ageing and infirmity confront us as the last part of life's drama unfolds before us. Christ is indeed the way, the truth and the life, and no one comes to a full knowledge of the Father except by traversing the way Jesus showed while he laboured with us. He was himself when he dined with sinners, and he was equally himself when he died between two of them on the cross. When his Father seemed furthest from him, separated from his consciousness by the miasma of human sin which he took unconditionally upon himself, he was closer both to us and to the Father than at any other time during his ministry among us.

It is our privilege to enjoy the fruits of health in order that we may be more profitable servants in the manifold activities of communal life in whatever situation we may find ourselves. And it is an even greater, if more awesome, privilege at the end of the day to be with Christ on the cross of human affliction, so that we, eternally in his company, can give an even greater support to those in need as we show the way forward. The way, which too is of Christ, leads through the darkness of mortal life to the effulgent splendour of the resurrection.

11

The Resurrection of the Body

There are heavenly bodies and earthly bodies; and the splendour of the heavenly bodies is one thing, the splendour of the earthly another. The sun has a splendour of its own, the moon another splendour and the stars another, for star differs from star in brightness. So it is with the resurrection of the dead. What is sown in the earth as a perishable thing is raised imperishable. Sown in humiliation, it is raised in glory; sown in weakness, it is raised in power; sown as an animal body, it is raised as a spiritual body.

(1 Cor. 15:40–4)

The end of human existence is to make real the divine spark within so that man may transcend his animal limitations and come to share in the very being of God, to quote 2 Peter 1:4 once more. This does not imply a negative view of our animal inheritance, that it is bad and has to be expunged; it affirms the holiness of all matter as a sacrament to be handled with love and reverence. But whereas the animal creation is mutable and destined to deterioration and death, the spiritual promise is one of growth beyond the limitation of our animal nature so that we may know and experience the life of eternity.

The spiritual body of which St Paul speaks is not to be seen merely as a vestment for the soul separated from the physical body at the time of death, suddenly taking the place of that perishable thing. It is rather to be envisaged as something we are building up even now while we are actively engaged in the life of the world. Its bricks and mortar are the thoughts we discharge into the psychic atmosphere, the attitudes we bring with us in our daily work, and above all the depth and veracity of relationship we create with those around us. According to the outgiving service and love we bestow on others – indeed on life itself – so is the spiritual body fashioned and refined. The more enclosed and selfish our ideals and attitudes and the more predatory our relationships with others, the more imperfect and threadbare is the spiritual body we are forming unobtrusively day by day, until the time that night comes when we can do no further work.

The purpose of spiritual healing is to open the portals of the personality to the full impact of the Holy Spirit so that what was once shuttered and isolated can now be brought to face the spiritual light of God. In one instance this opening of the personality to reality may be effected by a remarkable physical healing, such as the many wrought by Jesus during his ministry among us. On other occasions a dramatic mental healing may be the precursor of a complete change in outlook on life. The miracles of deliverance reported in the Gospel come into this category of mental renewal, remembering that possession is at most an added focus of disturbance in an already deranged personality. The prophecy of Isaiah 61:1–2 is the quintessence of all healing: bringing good news to the humble, binding up the broken-hearted, proclaiming liberty to captives, releasing the prisoners, proclaiming a year of the Lord's favour and comforting the mourner.

These manifold works that are the heart of true healing are performed by proclaiming the word of God, which is given to us when we are in attentive contemplation by the Holy Spirit, and then living that Word in our own lives. We remember that the name of the Word, when it became flesh and dwelt among us, was Jesus. The Christ life in us brings us close to the Holy Spirit, who transfigures in turn all who are disordered and stultified, so that they too come to be manifest sons of God, in something of the likeness of the Son of God, Jesus Christ. The good news for the humble is that the kingdom of God is here, so that the hearts of all who are available to give themselves to Him are filled with His Spirit.

The broken-hearted are restored by the ever-present love of God and inspired by the vision of a completeness of love that embraces all people; in this way their immediate, scarcely bearable tragedy is illuminated by a universal fellowship of all people living the life of Christ. The captives are liberated from the prison of their own minds, the walls of which are the unconscious elements of previous experiences as yet submerged and unassimilated. The radiant light of God's compassion enlightens these dark places of the soul, exposing invidious complexes to the blaze of full understanding, and then healing them. The Lord's favour is proclaimed by the healing powers that emanate from his ministers, so that the healing energies dormant in all people may be activated and blessed through the intercession of those who serve God in this great ministry. The mourner is comforted by the intimate communion he is granted with the beloved on the other side of death. This is a spontaneous, completely unpremeditated awareness of the unity of all life that is conveyed by the beloved in his new understanding acquired in the life beyond death. In this unity of life we are all, potentially at least, members of the Communion of Saints, and death is put in its proper perspective as an experience of transition from a limited, ego-centred type of consciousness to a more embracing fellowship with many people in a soul-centred consciousness. Here love is the centre and end of existence.

All life is punctuated by little deaths, in which the certainties of the past are rudely and irreversibly disrupted by a new event of the present. In adapting ourselves to the demands of the moment at hand, we learn with great alacrity to jettison old ways of thinking and to enter into a new mode of existence. By the time we come to spiritual maturity, at least in this world, we grasp the essential truth that we own nothing here at all. Our possessions are here to help us grow into more caring, responsible people – whether these possessions be material, intellectual or even relationships with other people whom we sincerely believe we love – but at the final death of this earthly life we have only ourselves with the spiritual body which has been assiduously constructed on the experiences of that life. As we are at the end, so we shall start in the new life ahead of us, but without a physical body under which

111

our baser emotions and more shady intentions can be hidden. 'We brought nothing into the world; for that matter we cannot take anything with us when we leave, but if we have food and covering we may rest content' (1 Tim. 6:7–8). The food of life is to work to God's honour and glory and the benefit of those around us; the covering is the spiritual body which will outlast all the vicissitudes of this life and be with us in the life beyond death.

There comes a time in the healing process when the person can be prepared to make the final renunciation. 'Abba, Father, all things are possible to thee; take this cup away from me. Yet not what I will, but what thou wilt' (Mark 14:36). These great words of Christ heralded his supreme healing work for humankind, the assumption of all human dread and humiliation, so that the full burden could be resurrected into the light of a greater forgiveness and understanding. While it is right that we should strive for healing of the physical body and mind in this world so long as it is yet day, there comes the night when work is finished and we have to submit in patient trust to the processes of transition to a greater life than we can as yet grasp. This applies not only to those who are terminally ill after having engaged in a prolonged, heroic fight against mounting adversity, but also those whose lives have been thwarted from birth because of irremediable physical or mental handicap. In the mute waiting that attends these tragic episodes the soul grows into a nobility of compassion that is often denied the activist in all his social concern. This growth of the soul into ultimate compassion applies not only to the afflicted one but also to those who attend him and watch with pained impotence his decline and death. We have to learn that healing is completed only when we can give of ourselves unconditionally to God's service, whose nature is constructive and whose end is a loving restoration of all things in the divine image, an image revealed definitively in Christ.

In the glorious resurrection of Jesus it would appear that even his tortured physical body was miraculously changed, so that it too contributed its quota to the spiritual body in which he revealed himself subsequently to the disciples. To the modern mind such a transmutation of coarse, perishable material elements to spiritual radiance seems beyond belief, and indeed is outside the scope of such scientific under-standing as we can at present muster. But the tradition, recorded faithfully in all four gospels, stands, and we would be wise to respect it even if we cannot fathom its mechanism in the current state of our knowledge. The phenomenon of spiritual healing, in which a dramatic physical change may follow closely on prayer or the laying-on of hands, does point to a mutability of the outer body that is not generally conceded in the obtuse mental climate of everyday life. The body, closely connected as it is with the mind and emotions, is in all probability less solid and more subject to subtle changes than is generally assumed. Studies in psychosomatic medicine and psychical phenomena are shedding increasing light on the plastic nature of matter generally and of the physical body in particular. If nuclear power is the result of a destructive conversion of matter to energy, it may transpire that spiritual healing is the result of a constructive effect of energy on living matter which is raised to a heightened potentiality of function and response. This energy is essen-tially psychic in nature, emanating from the living vibrancy of the soul. In St Paul's great mystical vision of Romans 8:21, the entire universe is to be freed from the shackles of mortality to enter upon the liberty and splendour of the children of God.

These thoughts must necessarily remain tentative in our present state of knowledge, but the well-attested phenomena of paranormal healing make them at least worthy of serious consideration. The material universe is indeed a sacrament of God's unceasing providence to His creatures, and it too has an eternal place in the divine economy. Quoting St Paul once more, this time in the context of the passage that prefixed this chapter, when death is swallowed up in victory, the perishable thing will be raised up imperishable, not only on a personal level, but also on a cosmic scale. Such, at any rate, is the promise of universal redemption in Christ. Admittedly our own physical bodies are to return to the dust of the earth from whose elements they were initially fashioned. But at the time of the Lord's second coming, to which all the great religious traditions, in their own way, look forward, it may

well be that the dust of the earth will itself be fully spiritualized in the way indicated by the change in Christ's own
physical body. It is certain that flesh and blood can never
possess the kingdom of God, and the perishable cannot
possess immortality (1 Cor. 15:50). St Paul at this point
expounds a 'mystery' of sudden transmutation, which is in
fact a common factor in all mystical experience. At once the
mortal life opens up into eternity, which is not a never-ending
time sequence but rather a state of being beyond the confines
of space and time in which all creatures are in union with
God and with each other. At last they realize their unique
nature when they have relinquished themselves entirely to life
in the power of love. They are now authentically parts of the
one body, whose nature is Christ himself (1 Cor. 12:27). It
is then that the end comes, when Christ delivers up the
kingdom to God the Father, after abolishing every kind of
domination, authority and power (1 Cor. 15:24). On one level
this can easily be dismissed as mere ecstatic exuberance, but
on a deeper note it is the end to which the whole created
universe moves, as is glimpsed in supreme mystical
illumination.

These enriching thoughts furthermore serve to remind us
that a full bodily resurrection is not merely an individual
event; it is above all communal and finally universal. It
involves a renewal of human society, the whole living world
which we use so carelessly and treat so shabbily, and ultimately the entire cosmos. Therefore the ministry of healing
cannot exclude aesthetics, remembering the powerful effect
for good or ill that music, the plastic arts and literature have
on the human psyche. Nor is the healing of the world oblivious
of economics, politics and the conservation of the earth's
resources. This does not imply that any particular economic
theory or political party is the right one, but the Spirit of
God must infuse and transfigure all theories and parties so
that they may radiate love and reconciliation where at present
there is intransigence, intolerance and hatred. We have to
learn the supreme lesson of Christ of loving our enemies and
praying for our persecutors (Mat. 5:44). This is neither easy
nor can it be contrived mechanically, like the ritual worship
devoid of a living relationship with God and one's fellows

that was so vehemently denounced by the prophets of Israel, especially Amos and Isaiah. It requires nothing less than a self-giving unto death, if need be, for the sake of truth and righteousness, with the promise of resurrection granted by God himself – for there is no greater love than this, that a man should lay down his life for his friends (John 15:13). In this respect that which is evil serves to diminish the human personality, enslaving it to the predatory will of a power-hungry individual often hiding beneath a plausible ideology. By contrast, the good inspires the human personality with the vision of God in whose service alone there is perfect freedom, because in that service the personality is transfigured from splendour to splendour into his likeness; this is the influence of the Lord who is Spirit, to quote for the last time from 2 Corinthians 3:18.

Love combats evil with the intention of saving those under its thraldom and ultimately transfiguring its energies so that they may be harnessed for constructive healing activity. When we give up our life for our friends, we remember, in accordance with the Parable of the Good Samaritan (Luke 10:29–37), that our friend is our immediate neighbour on the road of life, the stranger whom we encounter on our own road to Emmaus. Therefore Christ is in our neighbour, and is our neighbour also. He is our never-failing friend. Humanity is closer to ourself than our own superficial identity, and in Christ our humanity leads us to a knowledge of God himself. In Christ our humanity touches all life, indeed all creation. It is in dying for humanity in self-giving love that we raise all people to eternal life; and the risen human being starts the raising of all the creatures of the earth. 'In truth, in very truth I tell you, a grain of wheat remains a solitary grain unless it falls into the ground and dies; but if it dies, it bears a rich harvest' (John 12:24). This is the essence of an understanding of healing at its highest.

It follows that a true resurrection of the body finds its realization in the new man full of the Holy Spirit. There is a spiritualization of the rational mind, the emotions and the entire psychic life of the person. The healings of Jesus were something more than a restoration of a diseased part or organ to proper function so that the person could start to lead a normal life once more; they were also a sign that the kingdom of God was very near to the sufferer, and that the end of his travail, now so miraculously relieved, was that he should live the risen life, even the life of Christ: the life I now live is not my life, but the life which Christ lives in me, to quote Galatians 2:20 for the last time, as in the concluding bars of a great piece of music, the very symphony of life itself.

As Christ himself is a symbol of the common man in his glory and his agony, with the miraculous resurrection as the climactic culmination of the whole of human life, so the healings wrought by Jesus are true sacraments: outer and visible signs of an inner and spiritual grace. The end of the process is spiritual transfiguration, whereby the purely human now assumes something of the divinity in which it was originally conceived. The kingdom of God in everyday life is one of harmonious interaction between many different types of people, now restored to health and with a vision of reality that transcends mere selfish clinging and desire. Thus the outer manifestation of physical and mental healing presages the complete transformation of the human personality into something of the nature of God.